# Poisoning in the Modern World

*Edited by Ozgur Karcioglu*
*and Banu Arslan*

Published in London, United Kingdom

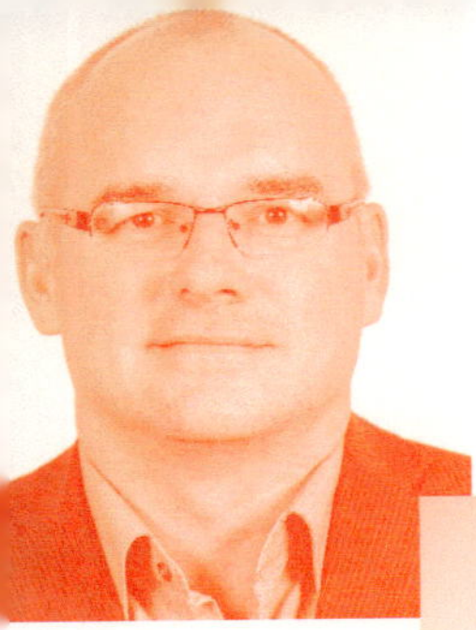
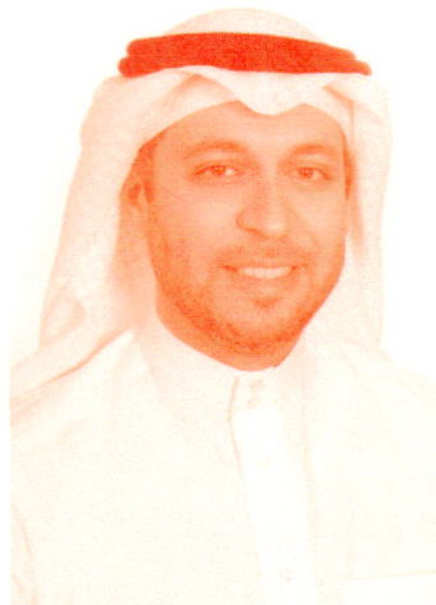
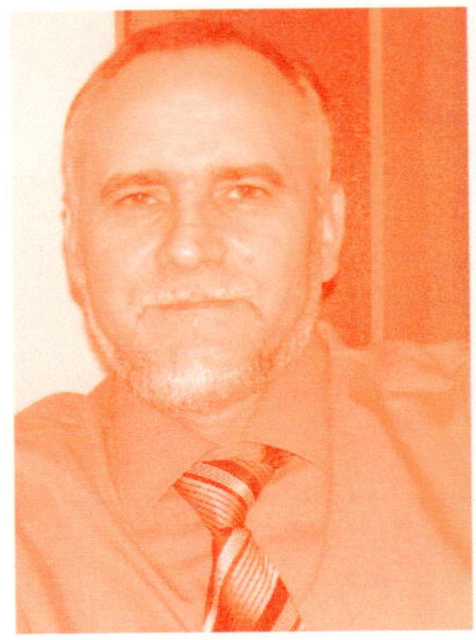
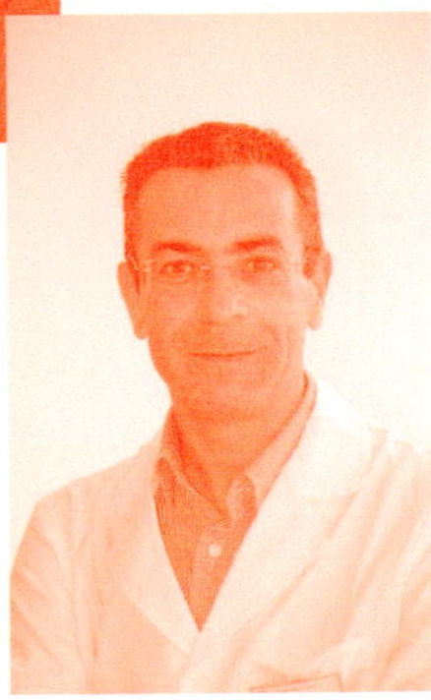
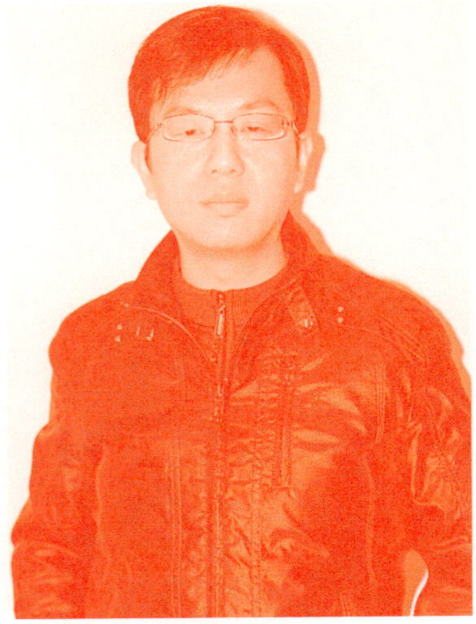
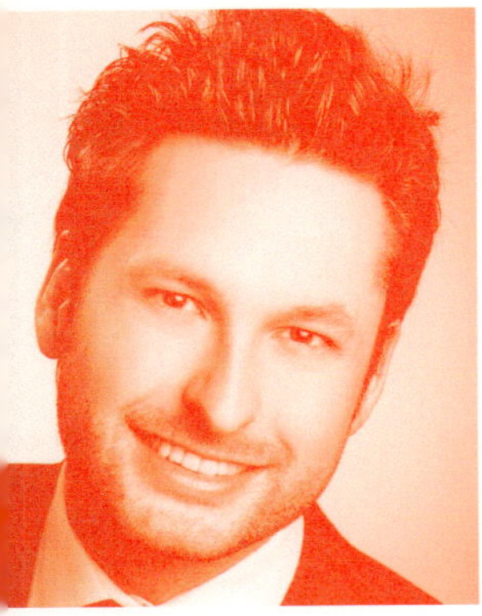
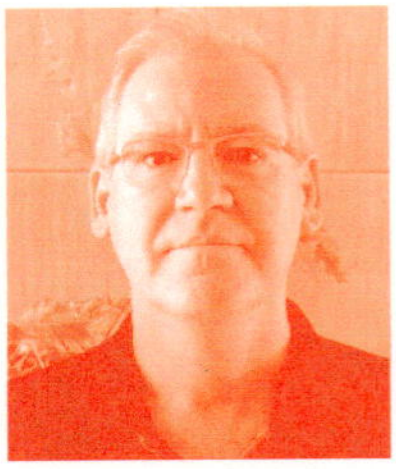

IntechOpen

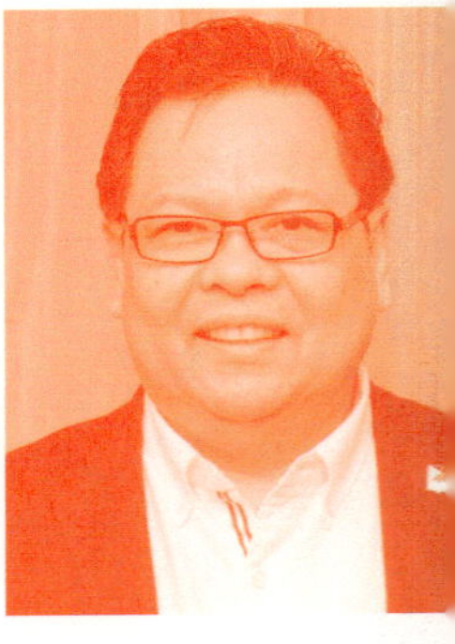
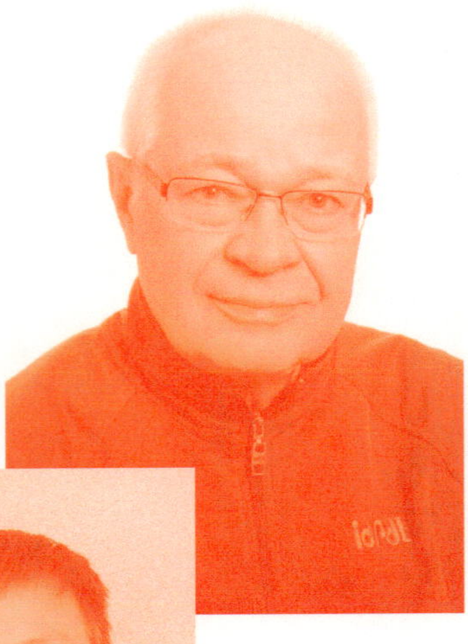
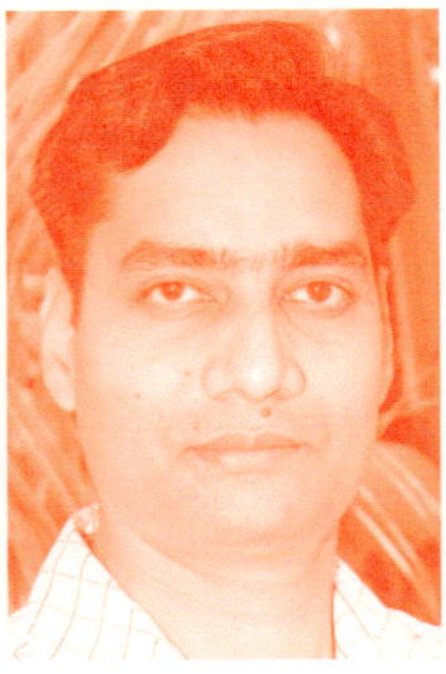
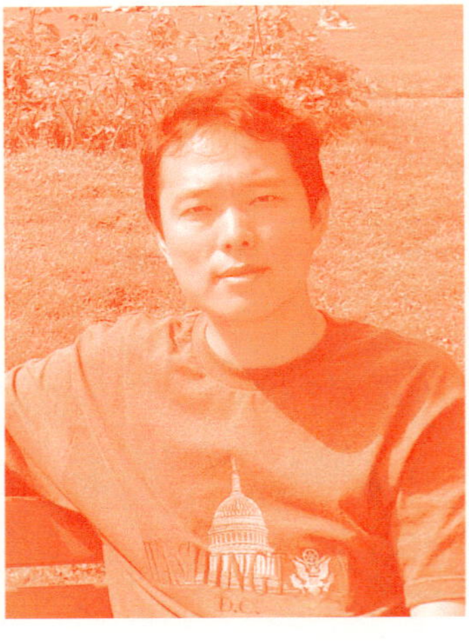
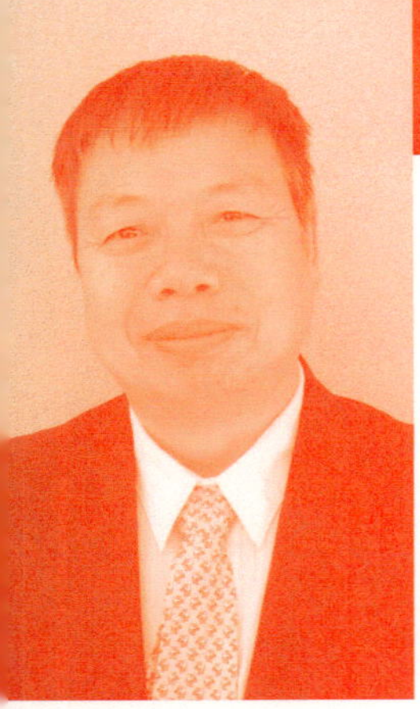
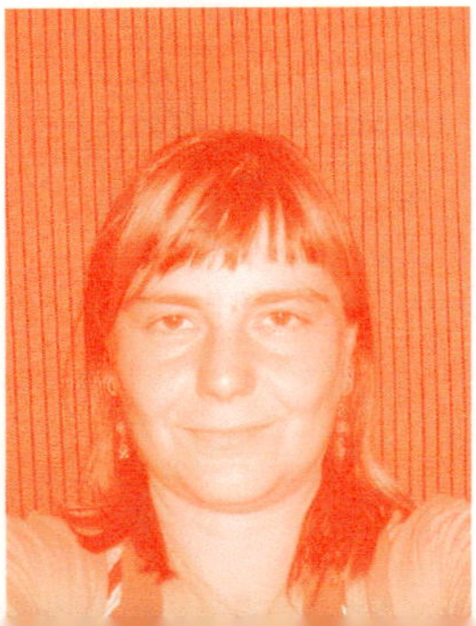

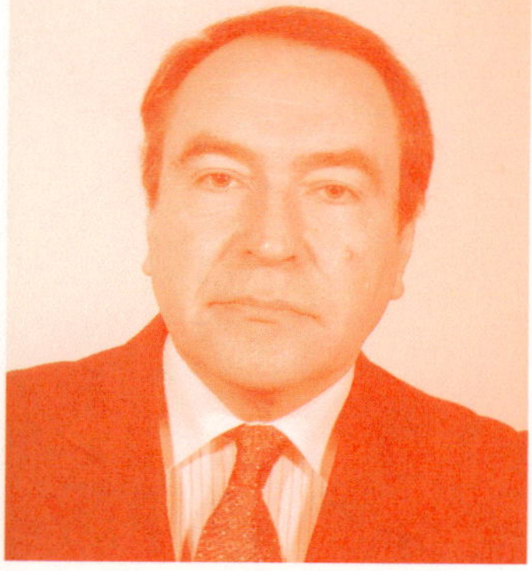
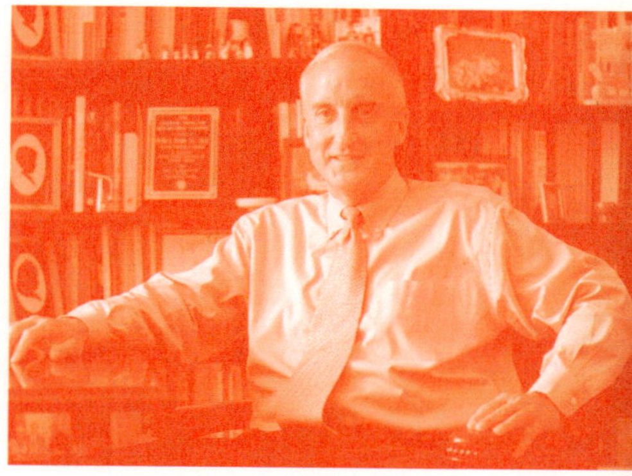
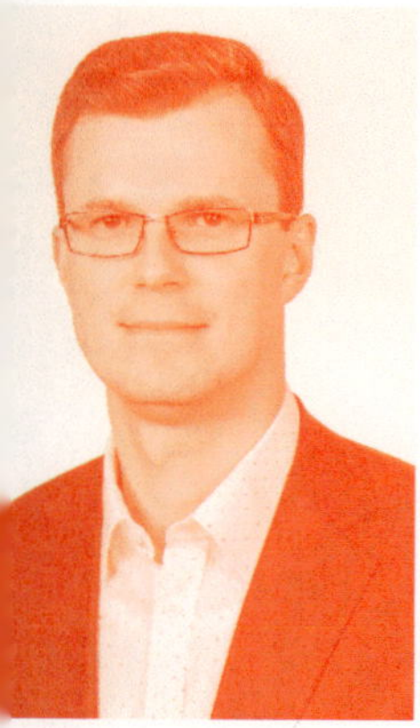
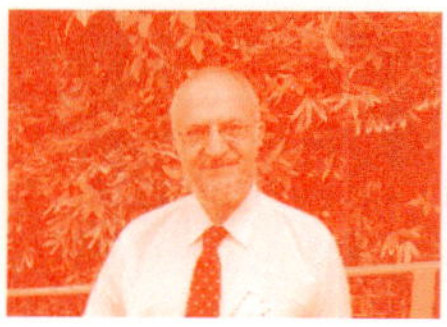
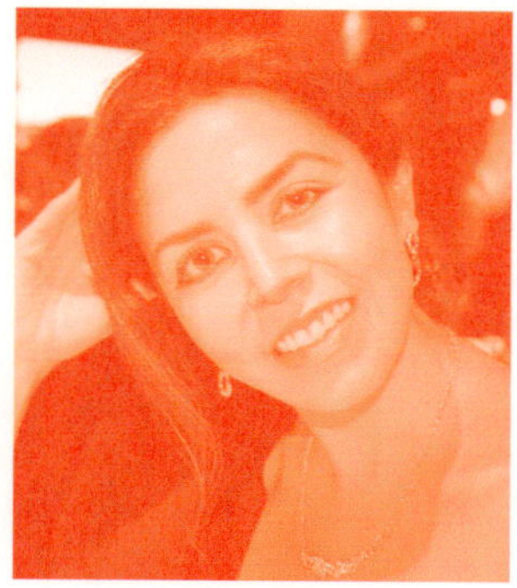

*Supporting open minds since 2005*

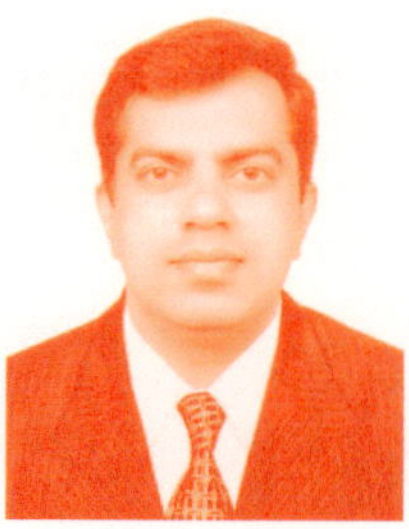
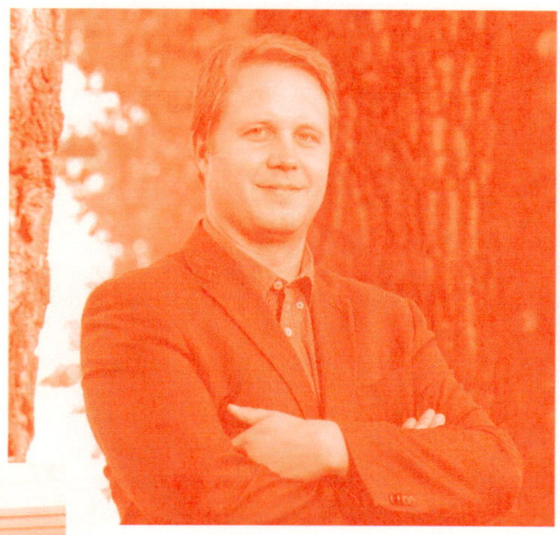
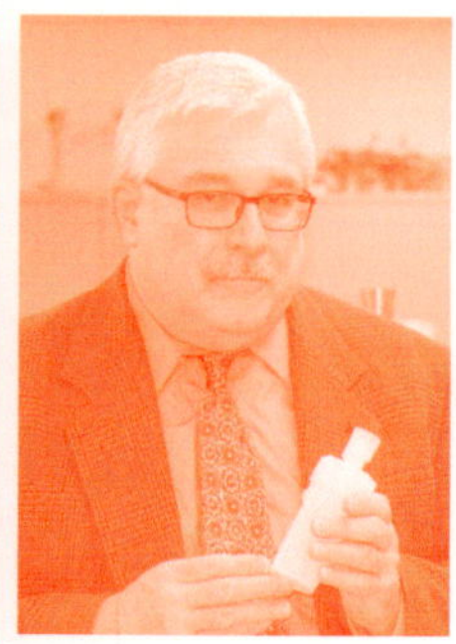
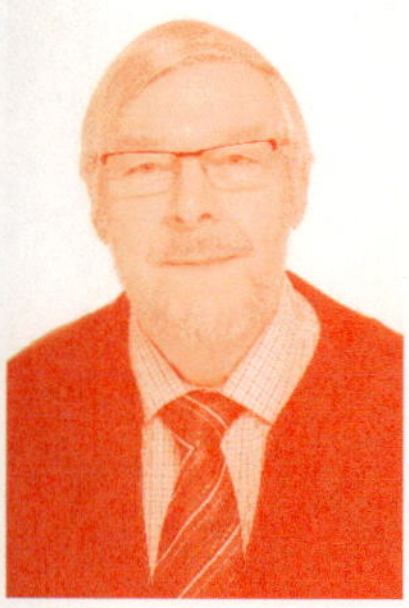
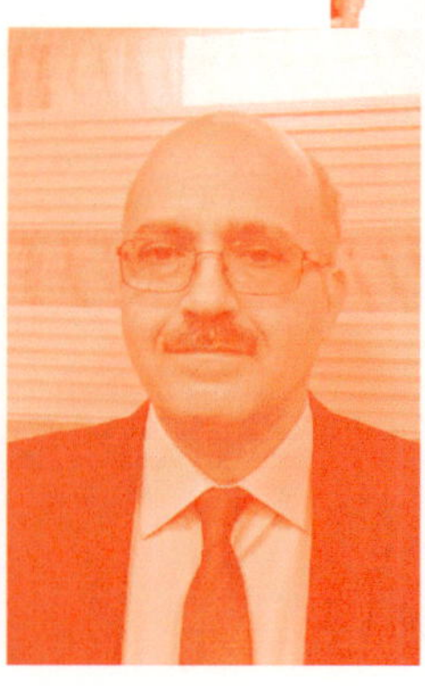
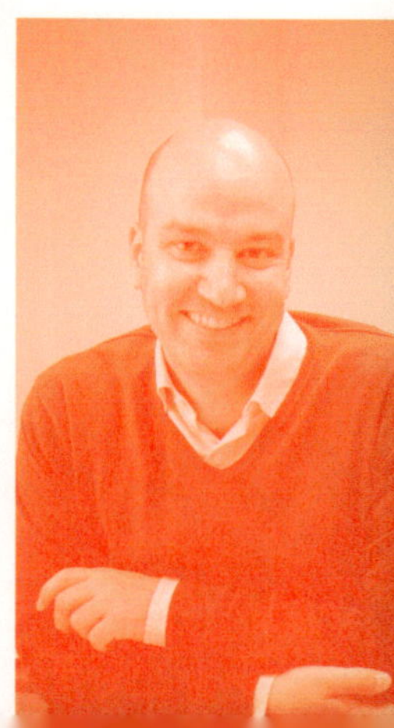
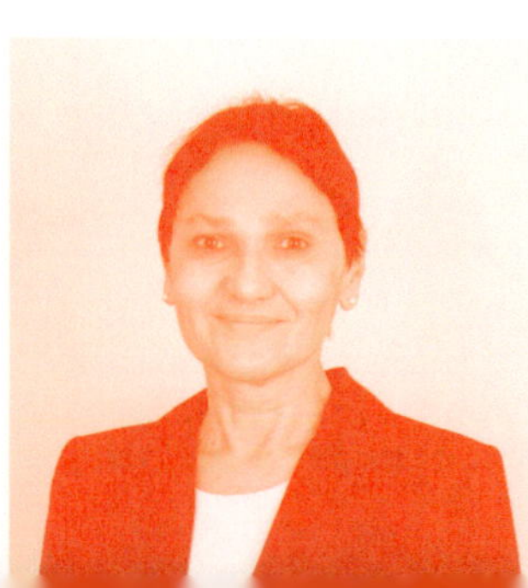

Poisoning in the Modern World
http://dx.doi.org/10.5772/intechopen.73906
Edited by Ozgur Karcioglu and Banu Arslan

Contributors
Sahar Issa, John Kanayochukwu Nduka, Azade Sari, Otilia Frasinariu, Nicolai Nistor, Irina Ciomaga, Aniela Rugina, Violeta Streanga, Ehab Aki, Godwill Azeh Engwa, Paschaline Ferdinand Okeke, Friday Nweke Nwalo, Marian Unachukwu



First published in London, United Kingdom, 2019 by IntechOpen
IntechOpen is the global imprint of INTECHOPEN LIMITED, registered in England and Wales, registration number: 11086078, The Shard, 25th floor, 32 London Bridge Street
London, SE19SG – United Kingdom
Printed in Croatia

British Library Cataloguing-in-Publication Data
A catalogue record for this book is available from the British Library

Additional hard and PDF copies can be obtained from orders@intechopen.com

Poisoning in the Modern World
Edited by Ozgur Karcioglu and Banu Arslan
p. cm.
Print ISBN 978-1-83880-785-6
Online ISBN 978-1-83880-786-3
eBook (PDF) ISBN 978-1-83880-787-0

For EU product safety concerns:
IN TECH d.o.o., Prolaz Marije Krucifikse Kozulić 3, 51000 Rijeka, Croatia, info@intechopen.com or visit our website at intechopen.com.

# Meet the editors

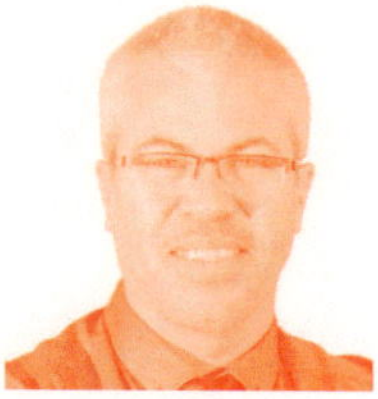

Dr. Ozgur Karcioglu, MD, graduated from residency in Dokuz Eylul University Medical School, Department of Emergency Medicine, Turkey, in 1998. He completed the "International Emergency Medicine" Fellowship in Penn State University in 2005. He now serves as the Chair of the Department of Emergency Medicine, Istanbul Education and Research Hospital. Dr. Karcioglu worked as a founder and board member of the Emergency Medical Association of Turkey after 1995. He has published more than 130 articles in scientific journals, contributed in 4 books as editor, and authored 35 chapters. Recently, he edited the book Trauma Surgery with the collaboration of IntechOpen. He is also an instructor of the Advanced Cardiac Life Support Course.

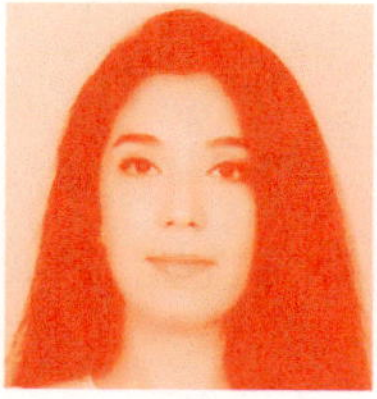

Dr. Banu Arslan, MD, MS, completed her emergency medicine residency at the University of Health Sciences, Istanbul Education and Research Hospital, in 2015. She worked at Kiziltepe Government Hospital, Mardin, from 2015 to 2016 where she gained experience in combat injuries and trauma care. She attended an Academic English Program at Southern Methodist University, TX, USA, between 2016 and 2017. Dr. Arslan worked as an attending emergency medicine physician, involved in teaching and clinical activities at Marmara University, Pendik Education and Research Hospital, from 2017 to 2018. Currently, she is studying MS in Healthcare Management at the University of Texas at Dallas. She has current certifications in ATLS, ACLS, and PALS. Her research interests are trauma care, toxicology, and healthcare financial management.

# Contents

# Preface

The term "poison" was first used in ancient French literature dating back to the Thirteenth century. Poisoning is a process in which an organism becomes severely chemically harmed by a toxic substance or venom. Poisoning, or the hazardous effects of foreign substances on the metabolism, has long been recognized as one of the greatest threats to public health. Industrialization, urbanization, economics, changes in communication, and availability of toxic agents, including various medicines, are among many factors that have an impact on patterns of human poisoning in the modern era.

It is important to increase awareness of the risk factors for poisoning with different substances: e.g., illicit drugs, industrial exposure, warfare agents, foods, and prescribed medicines, all of which can threaten an organism's homeostasis permanently or temporarily. On the other hand, standard medical education encompasses only a small part of toxicology and gives just a hint of how to manage a poisoned patient. Another point of view suggests that the importance of poisoning mandates a variety of clinicians, including almost all disciplines in medicine, namely, family physicians, emergency medicine physicians, pediatricians, and internists, who all have advanced knowledge of the management of poisoned patients.

Therefore, this book is intended for clinicians in routine practice who are willing to reach the contemporary literature data on different scenarios of poisoning and new techniques developed for elimination, decontamination, and treatment.

**Ozgur Karcıoglu, MD, FEMAT**
Professor,
Department of Emergency Medicine,
University of Health Sciences,
Istanbul Education and Research Hospital,
Fatih, Istanbul

**Banu Arslan, MD, MS**
Naveen Jindal School of Management,
Healthcare Management and Leadership Program,
University of Texas at Dallas,
USA

## Section 1

# General Principles in the Management of Intoxications

Chapter 1

# General Approach to Poisoned Patient

*Ehab Said Aki and Jalal Alessai*

## Abstract

Poisoning is a serious worldwide public health problem. Based on the World Health Organization data in 2012, almost 190,000 people died worldwide and the number of deaths due to poisoning in 2008 exceeded the number of deaths due to motor vehicular crashes; also, poisoning death rate nearly tripled worldwide. The number of patients presenting to the emergency departments with overdose had been increased both intentionally and accidentally. All the previous facts make toxicology an important field in emergency medicine. According to the American Association of Poison Control Centers (AAPCC) in the United States, over 2.1 million human exposure calls are reported in 2016. Management of intoxicated patients has a unique approach because of the challenge in diagnosis and treatment of overdose cases. This chapter focuses on general approaches for intoxicated patients and initial management and on how the history and physical examinations could help physicians to have a clue about the drugs that have been abused. Patients are most commonly poisoned via oral ingestion, but other routes could also cause intoxication including inhalation, insufflation, cutaneous and mucous membrane exposure, and injection.

**Keywords:** initial approach, physical examination, toxidromes, decontamination, toxicology laboratory

## 1. Introduction

Poisoning is a serious worldwide public health problem. Based on the World Health Organization (WHO) data in 2012, almost 190,000 people died worldwide and the number of deaths due to poisoning in 2008 exceeded the number of deaths due to motor vehicular crashes; also, the death rate due to poisoning nearly tripled worldwide. The number of patients presenting to the emergency departments with overdose had been increased both intentionally and accidentally. All the previous facts make toxicology an important field in emergency medicine [1, 2]. According to the American Association of Poison Control Centers (AAPCC) in the United States, over 2.1 million human exposure calls are reported in 2016.

Management of intoxicated patients has a unique approach because of the challenge in diagnosis and treatment of overdose cases. This chapter focuses on general approaches for intoxicated patients and initial management, explaining how the history and physical examinations could help physicians to have a clue about the drugs that have been abused. Patients are most commonly poisoned via oral ingestion, but other routes like inhalation, insufflation, cutaneous and mucous membrane exposure, and injection could also cause intoxication.

## 2. General approach to toxicological cases in emergency medicine

The approach to poisoned patients must be systematic. The range of symptoms and clinical findings in the physical examination are wide in drug poisoning patients; initial management is focused on stabilization of life-threatening conditions. The approach for the poisoned patients in emergency includes: resuscitation, history, physical examination, and management.

Initial screening examination should be done on all patients to find out immediate abnormal measures which need to be stabilized starting with vital signs, conscious level and pupil size, skin temperature, pulse oximetry, and electrocardiogram. Patients who are hemodynamically unstable must be kept in continuous cardiac monitoring. Intravenous access should be done and the blood glucose must be checked especially if the patients have a decreased level of consciousness.

## 3. Resuscitation

### 3.1 Airway and ventilation

The initial priorities for a poisoned patient presented to the emergency department are: securing the airway and breathing and stabilizing the circulation. Adequate ventilation and intubation with mechanical ventilation must be done early in the intoxicated patients with depressed mental status, except in cases of easy reversible causes of coma like opioid intoxication or hypoglycemia to prevent complications of intubation like aspiration. Other indications for intubation include severe acid-base disturbances or acute respiratory failure. In intubated patients, development of a respiratory acidosis must be prevented by adequate ventilation; in some cases like high-grade physiologic stimulation, the patient may need sedation and paralysis to prevent complications such as hyperthermia, acidosis, and rhabdomyolysis.

### 3.2 Hypotension

Drugs cause hypotension by four major mechanisms: decreased peripheral vascular resistance, decreased myocardial contractility, dysrhythmias, and depletion of intravascular volume. First-line treatment of hypotension is IV fluid bolus (10 to 20 mL/kg); if hypotension is not responding to fluid, it may be necessary to add vasopressors such norepinephrine. Norepinephrine is better than dopamine.

### 3.3 Hypertension

Elevated blood pursues caused by CNS sympathetic overactivity, increased myocardial contractility or increased peripheral vascular resistance, or a combination.

The treatment of hypertension and agitated patients starts with sedatives such as benzodiazepines; if not responding for initial treatment and there is evidence of end-organ dysfunction, calcium-channel blocker is preferred treatment. The use of beta-blockers is not recommended in the case of sympathetic hyperactivity because it may cause unopposed alpha-adrenergic stimulation and intensified vasoconstriction.

**Ventricular tachycardia** occurs because of tricyclic antidepressant toxicity. Sodium bicarbonate is first line therapy. Types IA (e.g., procainamide), IC, and III antiarrhythmic agents may worsen cardiac conduction; hence, they are not recommended; also, using these agents could be potentially dangerous.

Magnesium sulfate can also be used in the case of drug-induced torsade de pointes and prolonged QT intervals on ECG.

Digoxin toxicity with life-threatening tachyarrhythmias or bradyarrhythmias should be treated with specific Fab fragments (Digibind).

### 3.4 Bradyarrhythmias

Treatment of bradyarrhythmias with hypotension starts with atropine and/or temporary pacing. Calcium, glucagon, or high-dose insulin are used in the case of calcium channel blocker or beta blocker intoxication.

### 3.5 Seizures

The best treatment of intoxicated patients with seizures is benzodiazepines; we may add barbiturates if necessary. Phenytoin is not recommended to control seizures in poisoned patients.

### 3.6 Severe hyperthermia

Elevated temperature (hyperthermia) due to drug toxicity (e.g., sympathomimetic overdose, serotonin syndrome, or neuroleptic malignant syndrome) must be treated aggressively to prevent complications like rhabdomyolysis, organ failure, and disseminated intravascular coagulation. Treatment of hyperthermia includes active cooling like ice water immersion; if active cooling is ineffective, the patient may need sedation, neuromuscular paralysis, and intubation.

Patients presenting with signs of opioid overdose (low Glasgow coma scale-GCS respiratory depression, meiosis) must be given naloxone (0.1–2.0 mg I.V) as soon as possible [3].

## 4. History

History of the present illness is very important and can be obtained from the patients if they are alert and conscious; although the history following intentional ingestion is often unreliable, which makes history taking very challenging especially if the patients are comatose or cannot give their history, in such situations, history can be taken from collateral information from family, friends, ambulance crew, or medical records looking for past psychiatry illness, previous history of suicide or drug abuse, chronic medication, etc.

History must include time, route of entry, quantity, intentional or accidental exposure, availability of drugs at home, and if any member of the family has chronic diseases (hypertension, diabetic, etc.) and missing tablets or any empty pill bottles or other material was found around him [4]. It is very important to ask specifically about the use of traditional or herbal remedies and dietary supplements.

## 5. Physical examination

Physical examination of poisoned patients may give clues regarding the substance which has been abused and toxidromes. Physical examination includes: general appearance,

- Mental status (agitated or confused)

Some drugs or substances affect the central nervous system either causing agitation or depression.

Central nervous system depression may be caused by the following:

Anticholinergics, antidepressants, antipsychotics, lithium, cholinergic beta blockers, clonidine, and sedative-hypnotics.

Central nervous system agitation

Sympathomimetics, anticholinergics, salicylates, central hallucinogens, drug withdrawal states, carbon monoxide, hypoglycemic agents, and heavy metals.

- Skin (cyanosis, flashing, and physical signs of intravenous drug abuse (track marks)

Red and flushed skin occurs in the case of overdose of anticholinergic agents, antihistamines, TCAs, atropine, scopolamine, and phenothiazines.

Pale and diaphoretic skin occurs in the case of sympathomimetics (cocaine), cholinergic agents (organophosphates), central hallucinogens (lysergic acid diethylamide (LSD) and phencyclidine) and salicylate toxicities.

Cyanotic skin occurs in the case of methemoglobinemia and sulfhemoglobinemia.

- Eye examination: (pupil size reactivity lacrimation and nystagmus)

Common drugs causing miosis

- Opioids (morphine, hydromorphone, and oxycodone)
- Sedative-hypnotics (barbiturates and benzodiazepines)
- Cholinergic (nerve agents and organophosphate insecticides)
- Sympatholytic (clonidine and oxymetazoline)
- Common drugs causing mydriasis
- Sympathomimetics (cocaine and caffeine)
- Anticholinergics (atropine, scopolamine, and TCAs)
- Hallucinogens (LSD, mescaline, and psilocybin)
- Serotonin syndrome

Common drugs causing nystagmus
Barbiturates, carbamazepine, phencyclidine, phenytoin, and lithium

- Odor (garlic, bitter almonds, glue, alcohol, etc. (**Table 1**).
- Oropharynx hyper salivation or dryness;
- Chest: breath sound, bronchorrhea, wheezing, heart rate, and rhythm regularity;

| Substance | Odor |
|---|---|
| Ethanol, isopropyl alcohol, chloroform, salicylates | Acetone |
| Cyanide | Bitter almonds |
| Organophosphates, phosphorus | Garlic |
| Phosgene | Freshly mown hay |
| Hydrogen sulfide | Rotten eggs |

**Table 1.**
*Substances causing specific odor.*

- Abdomen examination (bowel sound, tenderness, and rigidity);
- Limbs (tremors and fasciculation), patient's clothing (looking for any medications and illegal drugs) [3].

### 5.1 Toxidromes

The term toxidrome was coined in 1970 by Mofenson and Greensher. Toxidromes are a group of abnormal physical examinations and abnormal vital signs known to be present with a specific group of medications or substances. The most common toxidromes are cholinergics, anticholinergics, sympathomimetics, opioids, and serotonin syndrome [4, 5].

### 5.2 Cholinergic toxidrome

Patients with cholinergic toxidrome present with wet manifestation. SLUDGE+3 Killer B′s and DUMBELLS are simple mnemonics for the common clinical symptoms. Also, patients present with bradycardia, hypertension or hypotension, tachypnoea, or bradypnea.

**SLUDGE:** salivation, lacrimation, urination, defecation, GI cramping, Emesis + Killer B′s: bronchorrhea, bradycardia, and bronchospasm.

**DUMBELLS:** diarrhea, urination, miosis (small pupils), bradycardia, emesis, lacrimation, lethargy, and salivation.

Most common causes: organophosphate pesticides, carbamates, some types of mushrooms, and sarin (warfare agent) [4].

### 5.3 Anticholinergic toxidrome

Patients present with anticholinergic toxidrome with dry manifestation, delirium, tachycardia, dry flushed skin, dilated pupils, hypertension, tachypnoea clonus, elevated temperature, decreased bowel sounds, and urinary retention. Simple mnemonics: "Hot as a Hare, Mad as a Hatter, Red as a Beet, Dry as a Bone, Blind as a Bat."

Most common causes: antihistamines, antiparkinsonians, atropine, scopolamine, amantadine, antipsychotics, antidepressants, muscle relaxants, and plants (jimsonweed) [4].

### 5.4 Sympathomimetic toxidrome

Patients present with CNS stimulation and psychomotor agitation, elevated blood pressure, tachycardia, dilated pupils, hyperthermia, widened pulse pressure, tachypnoea, hyperpnea diaphoresis, and seizure in severe cases.

Most common causes: cocaine and amphetamine.

### 5.5 Opioid toxidrome

The most common clinical presentation of opioid toxidrome are: coma, respiratory depression and meiosis, hypotension, hypothermia, bradycardia, and seizure that may occur in propoxyphene overdose, but small pupils not always present may present with normal size pupils such in meperidine and, propoxyphene toxicities [4].

### 5.6 Serotonin syndrome

Patients present with altered mental status, hypertensive, and tachycardia, myoclonus, hyperreflexia, hyperthermia, and increase in muscle rigidity. Most common causes: SSRI interaction or overdose of SSRIs.

MAOIs, tricyclic antidepressants, amphetamines, and fentanyl [4].

### 5.7 Neuromuscular malignant

Patients present with severe muscle rigidity, hyperpyrexia, altered mental status, autonomic instability, diaphoresis, mutism, incontinence. Most common causes: antipsychotic medication.

### 5.8 Sedative/hypnotic

Patients present with central nervous system depression, ataxia, dysarthria, bradycardia, respiratory depression, hypothermia, hypotension, and bradypnea. Most common causes are benzodiazepines and barbiturates.

### 5.9 Hallucinogenics

Patients present with hallucinations, perceptual distortions, depersonalization, synaesthesia, and agitation.

Mydriasis, hyperthermia, tachycardia, hypertension, tachypnoea, and nystagmus. Most common causes:

phencyclidine, LSD, mescaline, psilocybin, and MDMA ["Ecstasy"].

### 5.10 Ethanolic

Patients present with central nervous system depression, ataxia, dysarthria, and odor of ethanol.

### 5.11 Extrapyramidal

Patients present with dystonia, torticollis, muscle rigidity, choreoathetosis, hyperreflexia, and sometimes seizures. Most common causes: risperidone, haloperidol, and phenothiazines.

### 5.12 Salicylate

Patients with salicylate toxidrome present with altered mental status, mix respiratory alkalosis, metabolic acidosis, tinnitus, tachypnoea, tachycardia, diaphoresis, nausea, vomiting, and hyperpyrexia.

Most common toxin: aspirin and oil of wintergreen (methyl salicylate).

## 6. Management

### 6.1 Electrocardiogram (ECG)

ECG should be done on all patients who are symptomatic or who have been exposed to cardiotoxic agents looking for the rate and conduction; ECG abnormalities may help in diagnosis or may help as prognostic information. Specific attention should be paid to QRS interval and QT interval; in the case of prolongation of QT or QRS sodium bicarbonate infusion should be strongly considered.

### 6.2 Radiographic studies

Imaging examinations are not necessary in every poisoned patient but may be useful in some situations where the toxins are radiopaque [6]. The toxins which are radiopaque can be summarized by the mnemonic "CHIPES" (**Table 2**); also, "body packers" may be seen on plain films (**Figure 1**). Chest x-ray is useful in the case of noncardiogenic pulmonary edema and the acute respiratory distress syndrome due to exposure to certain toxins.

### 6.3 Abdominal ultrasound

Ultrasound abdomen is not helpful in poisoned patient and the use of ultrasound is very limited and does not appear to be a reliable method of detecting ingested toxins [7].

### 6.4 Laboratory test

Blood test must be done with all intoxicated patients; especially in the case of intentional overdose, the laboratory test should include basic lab (full cell count and kidney function liver function and electrolytes). Acetaminophen screening is very important in every patient presenting with altered mental status or intentional overdose [8].

For the patients with an acid-base abnormality, serum osmolarity needs to be checked, looking for increasing osmolar gap, which rolls out toxic alcohol ingestion.

In the case of presence of anion gap, metabolic acidosis may help and give to physician a clue of ingestion of certain toxins like (salicylates, ethylene glycol, and methanol or other drugs which may cause high anion gap metabolic acidosis; also serum creatinine, glucose, ketones, and lactate should be tested to detect other causes of the anion gap acidosis.

| C | **Chlorinated hydrocarbons, calcium salts, and crack vials** |
|---|---|
| H | Heavy metals (iron, arsenic, mercury, thallium, and lead) |
| I | Iodinated compounds (e.g., thyroxine) |
| P | Packets of drugs ("body packers"), Play-Doh potassium salts, psychotropics (e.g., phenothiazines, lithium, and cyclic antidepressants |
| E | Enteric-coated tablets (aspirin) |
| S | Salicylates, sodium salts, and sustained-release drugs |
| | Sustained-release preparations |

**Table 2.**
*Radiopaque toxins.*

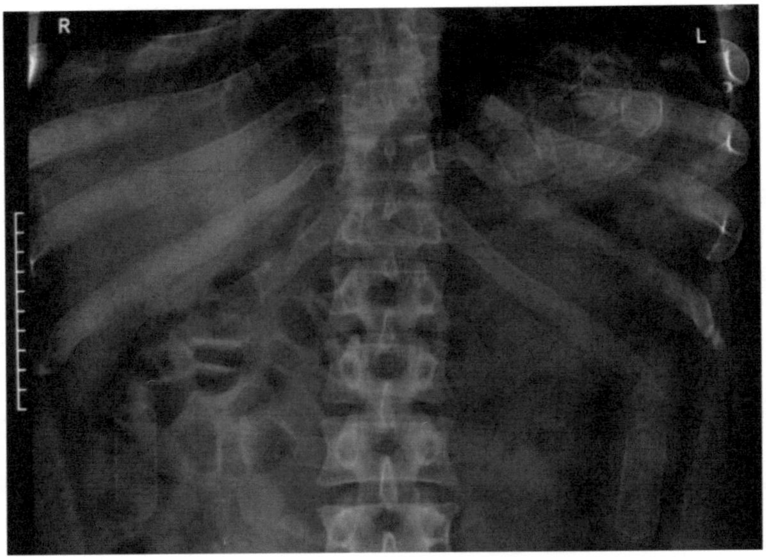


**Figure 1.**
*Body packers.*

When serum creatinine is elevated with a normal BUN, this finding is seen in the case of isopropyl alcohol toxicity (or with diabetic ketoacidosis). Co-oximetry can be used for rapid diagnosis of carbon monoxide toxicity and methemoglobinemia.

## 6.5 Toxicology screening

Toxicology screening is not necessary in case of nonintentional ingestion are asymptomatic patient or have clinical findings that are match with the medical history.

Drugs of abuse to opioids, benzodiazepines, cocaine metabolites, barbiturates, tricyclic antidepressants, tetrahydrocannabinol, and phencyclidine can be detected by using immunoassay screens in urine.

Positive and negative screens for drugs do not necessarily confirm diagnosis of acute poisoning but require further investigations.

## 6.6 Limitations of toxicologic drug screening assays

- Nonspecific—because most tests can detect only typical drugs within a class: opioids, amphetamines, benzodiazepines, cannabinoids, cocaine, barbiturates. For example, opioid screens do not detect meperidine and amphetamine screens do not detect methylenedioxymethamphetamine

- Drugs may be detected days to weeks after exposure. A positive test may not mean acute poisoning

- Cross reactivity in the case of carbamazepine, cyproheptadine, and chlorpromazine; the test can be positive for tricyclic antidepressants

- Test can be negative if tested urine was diluted.

## 7. Decontaminations

Decontamination of poisoned patient means removing the patient from the toxin and removing the toxin from the patient, either outside the patient's body by gross washing or inside the body by gastrointestinal decontamination or enhanced elimination.

### 7.1 Gross decontamination

Patient must be fully undressed and washed thoroughly with copious amount of water twice regardless of how much time has elapsed since the exposure. All the clothing must be removed and placed in plastic bags, and then the bags must be sealed; no need to neutralize an acid with a base or a base with an acid because that may lead to more tissue damage because the heat could be generated by this reaction. Using any greases or creams must be avoided because they will only keep the xenobiotic in close contact with the skin and ultimately make its removal more difficult.

Decontamination must be done in an isolated specific area. Gross decontamination is used in chemical, biological, and radiation exposure. Healthcare providers must wear universal precautions (gown, gloves, and eye protection) and sometimes may need personal protective equipment.

### 7.2 Ocular decontamination

In the case of eye exposures to chemical substance, initially, application of a local anesthetic agent (e.g., 0.5% tetracaine) may be needed, then copious irrigation with crystalloid solution. Lid retraction facilitates the irrigation. Alkalis cause more injury than acids because of deep tissue penetration via liquefaction so may need prolonged irrigation (1 to 2 hours). pH of conjunctival sac should be tested and irrigation should be continued until pH is <7.4.

### 7.3 Gastrointestinal decontamination

There are multiple methods used for gastrointestinal decontamination including:

- Emesis

Induced vomiting by ipecac syrup can decrease absorption and was used in the past but now is rarely indicated because there is no evidence supporting its effectiveness in reducing toxin absorption. It may also increase the risk of complications. Syrup ipecac may be considered in conscious, alert patients with ingestion of a potential number of toxic drugs and present in a very short time after ingestion (<1 hour).

Contradictions:

- Unprotected airway
- Corrosive/hydrocarbon ingestion
- Unstable patient status (hypotensive-seizure) [9].
- Gastric lavage

Gastric lavage is an intervention widely used to remove the ingested toxin drugs from the stomach by an orogastric tube. Because of the absence of published evidence that shows that orogastric lavage may change the outcome, now orogastric lavage is rarely indicated. It may be considered in the case of recent (<1 hour) ingestion of life-threatening amount of a toxin for which there is no effective treatment once absorbed.

Contraindications:

- Corrosive/hydrocarbon ingestion
- Supportive care/antidote likely to lead to recovery
- Unprotected airway
- Unstable, requiring further resuscitation (hypotension and seizures).

Complications:

- Aspiration pneumonia
- Water intoxication
- Hypothermia
- Laryngospasm
- Mechanical injury to gastrointestinal tract.
- Activated charcoal:

Activated charcoal is a super-heating carbonaceous material. Activated charcoal works by reducing the absorption of a substance in the gastrointestinal lumen but it is not effective in metal, alcohols, corrosives, and lithium. The most effective action can be achieved when activated charcoal is given within the first hour of ingestion. In the case of intubated patients, activated charcoal may be administered via an orogastric or nasogastric tube.

Dose:

- Children 1 to 12 years of age: 25 to 50 g or 0.5 to 1.0 g/kg (maximum dose 50 g)
- Adults: 25 to 100 g (with 50 g representing the usual adult dose).

Contraindications:

Substances not adsorbed by activated charcoal.

- Unprotected airway
- Corrosive ingestion
- Upper gastrointestinal perforation.

*DOI: http://dx.doi.org/10.5772/intechopen.84681*

Complications:

- Vomiting
- Aspiration of the activated charcoal
- Reduce absorption of orally administered antidotes [10]
- Whole-bowel irrigation:

Whole-bowel irrigation is a mechanical cleansing of the whole gastrointestinal track reducing toxin absorption. The whole-bowel irrigation can be done by Polyethylene glycol solution. Polyethylene glycol is an osmotically balanced electrolyte solution; polyethylene glycol can be given orally to cooperative, awake patients. Patient positioning (head up 30°) reduces the risk of pulmonary aspiration; during whole-bowel irrigation also bowel sounds must be present. Clear rectal effluent and imaging shows the absence of foreign bodies considered as endpoint of whole-bowel irrigation treatment.

Indication:

- Iron ingestion >60 mg/kg with opacities on abdominal radiograph
- Life-threatening ingestion of diltiazem or verapamil
- Body packers or stuffers
- Slow-release potassium ingestion
- Lead ingestion (including paint flakes containing lead)
- Symptomatic arsenic trioxide ingestion
- Life-threatening ingestions of lithium
- Contraindications
- Unprotected airway.

Gastrointestinal obstruction absent bowel sound or perforation [11].

Recurrent, unstoppable vomiting.

Complications:

- Nausea and vomiting
- Pulmonary aspiration
- Vomiting, bloating, and rectal irritation.

## 8. Enhanced elimination

Enhanced elimination is a method used to increase the rate of toxic removal from the body so as to reduce the severity and duration of clinical intoxication.

Enhanced elimination methods are not routinely used in poisoned patients. The indications for enhanced elimination include: [4].

- Severe toxicity
- Poor outcome despite supportive care/antidote
- Slow endogenous rate of elimination.

There are different techniques to enhance elimination:

**Multiple dose activated charcoal (MDAC).**

MDAC is defined as at least two sequential doses of activated charcoal [12]. Multidose activated charcoal can be given via orogastric or nasogastric tube to intubated patients.

Mechanism of action:

- Prevents ongoing absorption of toxin that persists in the GI tract (modified-release preparation)
- Enhances elimination in the post absorptive phase by delayed enterohepatic recirculation or enteroenteric recirculation ("gut dialysis").

Indications:

Ingestion of a life-threatening amount of carbamazepine, dapsone, phenobarbital, quinine, salicylates, or theophylline.

Ingestion of a life-threatening amount of another toxin that undergoes enterohepatic or enteroenteric recirculation and that is adsorbed to activated charcoal.

Ingestion of a significant amount of any slowly released toxin.

Contraindications:

- Unprotected airway
- Bowel obstruction.

Complications:

- Vomiting
- Pulmonary aspiration
- Constipation
- Bowel obstruction or perforation.

Dose: no optimal dose of MDAC has been established. But the acceptable regimen of 50 g is administered every 4 hours, or 25 g every 2 hours. Study on volunteer found no difference in effectiveness of larger doses spread out over time compared to smaller, more frequent dose [13].

- Urinary alkalinization

Urine alkalinization is a treatment regimen which enhances the elimination of toxins by administration of intravenous sodium bicarbonate to produce urine with pH > or = 7.5.

Alkaline urine acts on ionization of acidotic toxins within renal tubules, stopping resorption of the ionized drug back across the renal tubular epithelium and enhancing elimination through the urine [14].

Characteristics of drugs which respond to urinary alkalinization are [15].

- Eliminated predominantly unchanged by the kidney
- Distributed primarily in the extracellular fluid compartment
- Minimal protein-bound
- Weak acids (3.0 to 7.5).

Urinary alkalinization for poisoned patients can be done by the following steps:

- Correct hypokalemia
- Start with 1 to 2 mEq/kg IV sodium bicarbonate bolus
- Infuse 100 mEq of sodium bicarbonate mixed with 1 L of D5W at 250 mL/h
- Potassium chloride (20 mEq) can be added to maintain normokalemia
- Monitoring serum potassium and bicarbonate level every 2 to 4 hours to prevent hypokalaemia
- Urine pH should be checked regularly, keeping urine pH between 7.5 and 8.5.

Indications:

- Moderate to severe salicylate toxicity
- Phenobarbital severe toxicity
- Chlorophenoxy herbicide severe toxicity
- Chlorpropamide severe toxicity.

Contraindications:

- Pre-existing fluid overload
- Renal impairment
- Uncorrected hypokalaemia.

Complications:

- Hypokalaemia

- Volume overload
- Alkalemia.
- Urinary acidification (urine pH below 5.5) with ammonium chloride or ascorbic acid was used in the past to treat toxicity of weak bases such as amphetamines, quinidine, or phencyclidine. However, this practice is not used now because of lack of evidence of efficacy and complications such as iatrogenic toxicity (from severe academia) and rhabdomyolysis may occur.
- Extracorporeal elimination includes hemodialysis, hemoperfusion, and continuous renal replacement therapies, this method has limited indications in intoxicated patients, extracorporeal elimination need critical care setting also this procure are expensive and invasive, are not always available extracorporeal elimination were used in less than 0.1% of cases reported to U.S. poison control centers in 2010 [16]. The toxins need to have a number of criteria to be effectively removed by extracorporeal elimination [17]:
- low volume of distribution (<1.0 L/kg),
- low molecular weight (<500 Da), relatively
- low protein binding
- low endogenous clearance.

Indications:
Life-threatening toxicity of

- Lithium
- Metformin lactic acidosis
- Phenobarbital
- Salicylates
- Valproic acid
- Methanol/ethylene glycol
- Potassium salts
- Theophylline.

Contraindications:

- Hemodynamic instability
- Active hemorrhage
- Severe thrombocytopenia
- Sever coagulopathy

## 9. Extracorporeal membrane oxygenation (ECMO)

**ECMO:** extracorporeal technique used when the patients are critically ill and they cannot provide an adequate amount of gas exchange or perfusion to sustain. This technique may be used in the case of severe and massive overdose especially cardiotoxic drugs (beta blockers, calcium channel blocker) [18].

## 10. Antidotes

Although supportive care is the main treatment of most poisoned patients, there are cases in which administration of a specific antidote is potentially life-saving. Antidote is a substance that can prevent further poisoning from specific substances. **Table 3** shows the most common antidote used in the emergency department (see **Table 1**) [4].

| Toxin | Antidote |
|---|---|
| Acetaminophen | N-acetylcysteine 150 mg/kg dextrose IV over 15–60 min, then 50 mg/kg NAC IV over 4 hrs. Then 100 mg /kg NAC IV over 16 hrs. |
| Cholinergic (organophosphates, carbamates) | Atropine 1-2 mg every 2–3 min, until there is drying of secretions, pralidoxime (2-PAM) 70 mg/kg IV, then infusion at 500 mg/hour |
| Anticholinesterases | Physostigmine 0.5–1 mg IV as a slow push over 5 min and repeated every 10 min |
| Benzodiazepines | Flumazenil 0.2 mg repeated; max dose: 2 mg |
| β-Blockers | Glucagon 3–10 mg |
| Calcium channel blockers | Calcium gluconate 10% 10–30 mL IV |
| Cyanide | Amyl nitrite, sodium thiosulfate, sodium nitrite (3% solution), and Vitamin B12 |
| Digoxin | Digoxin Fab 5–10 vials |
| Isoniazid | Pyridoxine (vitamin B6) 70 mg/kg IV (maximum 5 g) |
| Methanol, ethylene glycol | Ethanol loading: 8 ml/kg of 10% ethanol then 1–2 ml/kg/hour of 10% ethanol; fomepizole Loading: 15 mg/kg in 100 ml IV over 30 min. Maintenance: 10 mg/kg IV over 30 min every 12 hours for 48 hr. |
| Narcotics | Naloxone 0.1–0.4 mg, may be repeated |
| Tricyclic antidepressants | Sodium bicarbonate 1–2 mEq/kg IV bolus followed by 2 mEq/kg per h IV infusion |
| Iron | Deferoxamine IV infusion dose of 15 mg/kg/hour |
| Methaemoglobinaemia | Methylene blue 1–2 mg/kg (0.1–0.2 ml/kg of 1% solution) IV slowly over 5 min |
| Local anesthetics | Intravenous lipid emulsion 1–1.5 ml/kg 20% IV bolus over 1 min, repeat bolus at 3–5 min, then infuse 0.25 ml/kg/min |
| Wernicke's syndrome, wet beriberi | 100 mg IV |
| Insulin, oral hypoglycemics | Dextrose (glucose) 1 g/kg IV |

**Table 3.**
*Antidote.*

## 11. Disposition

If the patient has persistent and toxic effects, the patient will require prolonged care course. Admission is indicated for completing his treatment and observation; in the case of severe toxicity, the patient may need admission to intensive care unit.

In the case of mild toxicity or asymptomatic patient, a 6-hour observation period is sufficient to exclude the development of serious toxicity.

A number of toxins have delayed onset clinical toxicity, for example (but not limited to): modified-release preparations of calcium channel antagonists, selective norepinephrine reuptake inhibitors (tramadol and venlafaxine), and newer antipsychotics (amisulpride); this means that the duration of observation should be longer than usual.

The decision to admit a patient with a toxic exposure to an intensive care setting should be based upon clinical criteria that relate to the stability of the airway, respiratory system, cardiovascular system, and the patient's level of consciousness.

A retrospective study which was done in more than 200 patients with drug overdoses shows that clinical assessment in the emergency department could reliably find out patients who are at high risk for complications and need intensive care unit admission [19].

Based on the following clinical criteria: if the patient has one of any of the following clinical criteria, the patient may need admission to intensive care unit:

- $PaCO_2$ > 45 mmHg
- Intubated patient
- Seizures post-ingestion
- Unresponsiveness to verbal stimuli
- Abnormal cardiac rhythm (nonsinus)
- Atrioventricular block (Second- or third-degree)
- Systolic blood pressure below 80 mmHg
- QRS duration ≥0.12 seconds.

## 12. Conclusion

The first step in the approach to intoxicated patient should start with stabilization measures including protected airway and adequate ventilation and circulation and control of the convulsion.

History in poisoning cases could be difficult; especially in self-harm poisoning or comatose patients, the physician must use collateral information from friends, family, prehospital personal and medical records.

Always ask, especially about the use of over-the-counter drugs and traditional or herbal preparations.

Physical examination may help to find the toxidrome and complication of toxins; physical examination should include all systems.

Focused laboratory test helps physicians to understand the severity of toxicity and suspected toxin and guides in management, making sure the drug level is sent at proper time not so early or late to avoid wrong interpretation; urine or blood toxicology screen assays have limited value in the case of acute over dose. Most of poisoned patients only supportive care with decontamination will be sufficient for them, but antidotes same times is the cornerstone of the treatment.

In the end, remember all the time "treat the patient, not the poison."

## Author details

Ehab Said Aki* and Jalal Alessai
Emergency Department, Hamad Medical Corporation, Doha, Qatar

*Address all correspondence to: akiehab2004@gmail.com

## References

[1] Warner M, Chen LH, Diane M, Makuc RN, Anderson AM. Miniño. Drug poisoning deaths in the United States, 1980–2008. NCHS Data Brief. 2011;**81**:1-8

[2] Liu Q, Zhou L, Zheng N, et al. Poisoning deaths in China: Type and prevalence detected at the Tongji Forensic Medical Center in Hubei. Forensic Science International. 2009; **193**:88

[3] Erickson TB, Thompson TM, Lu JJ. The approach to the patient with an unknown overdose. Emergency Medicine Clinics of North America. 2007;**25**:249

[4] Shaun G. General management of poisoned patients. In: Tintinalli JE, et al., eds. Tintinalli's Emergency Medicine Comprehensive Study Guide. 8th ed. New York, NY: McGraw-Hill; 2016

[5] Mofenson HC, Greensher J. The nontoxic ingestion. Paediatric Clinics of North America. 1970;**17**(3):583-590

[6] Savitt DL, Hawkins HH, Roberts JR. The radiopacity of ingested medications. Annals of Emergency Medicine. 1987; **16**(3):331-339

[7] Taftachi F, Sanaei-Zadeh H, Zamani N, Emamhadi M. The role of ultrasound in the visualization of the ingested medications in acute poisoning—A literature review. European Review for Medical and Pharmacological Sciences. 2012;**16**(15):2175-2177

[8] Sporer KA, Khayam-Bashi H. Acetaminophen andsalicylate serum levels in patients with suicidal ingestion or altered mental status. The American Journal of Emergency Medicine. 1996; **14**(5):443-446

[9] Manoguerra AS, Cobaugh DJ. Guidelines for the Management of Poisoning Consensus Panel: Guideline on the use of ipecac syrup in the out-of-hospital management of ingested poisons. Clinical Toxicology (Philadelphia). 2005;**43**:1

[10] Adams BK, Mann MD, Aboo A, et al. Prolonged gastric emptying half-time and gastric hypomotility after drug overdose. The American Journal of Emergency Medicine. 2004;**22**:548

[11] Lheureux P, Tenenbein M. Position paper: Whole bowel irrigation. Journal of Toxicology. Clinical Toxicology. 2004;**42**(6):843

[12] Vale JA, Krenzelok EP, Barceloux GD. Position statement and practice guidelines on the use of multi-dose activated charcoal in the treatment of acute poisoning. American Academy of Clinical Toxicology: European Association of Poisons Centres and Clinical Toxicologists. Journal of Toxicology. Clinical Toxicology. 1999;**37**:731-751

[13] Ilkhanipour K, Yealy DM, Krenzelok EP. The comparative efficacy of various multiple-dose activated charcoal regimens. The American Journal of Emergency Medicine. 1992;**10**(4):298

[14] Proudfoot AT, Krenzelok EP, Vale JA. Position paper on urine alkalinization. Journal of Toxicology: Clinical Toxicology. 2004;**42**:1-26

[15] Garrettson LK, Geller RJ. Acid and alkaline diuresis. When are they of value in the treatment of poisoning? Drug Safety. 1990;**5**:220

[16] Bronstein AC, Spyker DA, Cantilena LR Jr, et al. Annual report of the American Association of Poison Control Centers' National Poison Data System (NPDS): 28th annual report. Clinical Toxicology (Philadelphia). 2010, 2011; **49**:910-941

[17] Fertel BS, Nelson LS, Goldfarb DS. Extracorporeal removal techniques for the poisoned patient: A review for the intensivist. Journal of Intensive Care Medicine. 2010;**25**:139-148

[18] Rona R, Cortinovis B, Marcolin R, et al. Extra-corporeal life support for near-fatal multi-drug intoxication: A case report. Journal of Medical Case Reports. 2011;**5**:231. DOI: 10.1186/1752-1947-5-231

[19] Brett AS, Rothschild N, Gray R, et al. Predicting the clinical course in intentional drug overdose. Implications for use of the intensive care unit. Archives of Internal Medicine. 1987; **147**(1):133-137

Chapter 2

# Poisoning in the Pediatric Intensive Care Unit

*Nicolai Nistor, Otilia Frăsinariu, Aniela Rugină, Irina Mihaela Ciomaga and Violeta Ştreangă*

## Abstract

Poisonings during childhood (both accidental and voluntary) are a common cause of presentation in the emergency departments (EDs) and the pediatric intensive care unit (PICU). The admission to PICU is warranted both for treatment and for continuous monitoring, as sometimes the evolution of a poisoning could be unpredictable. Sometimes, complications arise that may prolong the patients' hospitalization and may contribute to lowering the survival rate. The staff in these departments must be well trained to ensure patient monitoring, early detection of complications, and rapid intervention. Supporting vital functions is the main objective of the management of a poisoned patient admitted in PICU. In recent years, staff competence and advanced medical technology have helped to improve the prognosis of the patients admitted to these departments, including of the poisoned patients.

**Keywords:** intensive care, poisoning, children

## 1. Introduction

Poisoning is a relatively common medical emergency worldwide and raises particular problems of diagnosis and treatment especially in children, regardless of the path the toxic enters the body (ingestion, inhalation, injection, or skin absorption). This age group is the most vulnerable population with the highest risk of accidental intoxications that can be partially prevented [1]. It is a common cause of presentation in the ED and the PICU. Early identification of the clinical characteristics of patients with acute intoxication and rapid initiation of therapy in these services can help reduce the mortality of intoxicated patients [2, 3]. These departments have the ability to continuously monitor vital parameters, use the most advanced medical technology and the most appropriate treatment. Usually, admission to PICU is by ED or by transfer from another hospital [4]. Often, a poisoned patient will be brought into intensive care not for treatment, but for continuous surveillance and monitoring in order to minimize mortality. On the other hand, care in these units has a very high cost. It is therefore recommended that the admission of poisoning cases in intensive care should take into account the efficient use of resources without compromising patient care [5]. The percentage of children with acute poisoning in PICU ranges from 8% [6] to 11.7% [2]. In the United States in 2014, 2336 intoxicated patients admitted to intensive care units needed ventilatory support, 509 received vasopressors, and 127 needed hemodialysis [4].


IntechOpen

## 2. Admission of intoxicated patients in PICU

There are several studies that attempt to establish criteria for admission to intensive care in patients based on severity scores (APACHE II/III, PRISM II/III, SAPS II, Glasgow etc.). These included patients with various medical and surgical conditions, but few can be validated using such scoring systems in poisoned patients [7–9]. Until more specific poisoning factors are established, it is thought that experience and proper clinical judgment can predict which patients will receive intensive care. The presence of certain abnormal symptoms or abnormal test results may require monitoring and/or treatment in PICU regardless of the suspected toxic. This approach is more consistent with the principle of "treating the patient and not the poison" [5]. It should be kept in mind that an initially asymptomatic poisoned patient may worsen later. Poisoned children and adolescents should be directed to the nearest intensive care unit that has pediatric critical care practitioners and equipment appropriate to pediatric age.

### 2.1 Criteria for admission to intensive care of the poisoned patient

I. Acute respiratory failure characterized by one or more of the following [4]:

- Need for ventilatory support or emergency tracheostomy.
- Marked respiratory compromise as indicated by:

  a. FR <20 or >60 for children <1 year and <12 or >60 for children >1 year.

  b. $SpO_2$ <92% when $O_2$ is administrated by mask or tracheostomy.

  c. $PaO_2$ <80 mm Hg at 100% $O_2$ administrated by mask.

- Rapidly progressive deterioration in respiratory status.
- Respiratory acidosis with $PaCO_2$ > 60 mmHg and pH < 7.25.
- Airway obstruction, apnea, anaphylaxis.

II. Hemodynamic instability or circulatory insufficiency characterized by one or more of the following:

- Shock as indicated by capillary refill time >4 s, distal or proximal nonpalpable pulse, systolic TA < lower age limit or TA < mean 50 mmHg (<40 mmHg in newborn), metabolic acidosis with < pH 7.25, base deficit >10 or serum bicarbonate <10 mEq/l, need for invasive hemodynamic monitoring.
- Cardiac instability and arrhythmia, necessity of continuous perfusion or vasoactive substances, ECG ischemic changes, congestive heart failure, and vascular volume instability.

III. Neurological instability manifested by one or more of the following:

- Neurological damage with one or more of the following: Glasgow score <10, severe irritability, hallucinations, and change of posture.
- Intracranial bleeding, increased intracranial pressure, seizures, or delirium.

IV. Severe metabolic disorders: serum Na <125 mmol/l or >160 mmol/l, serum K <3 mmol/l or >6.5 mmol/l, glucose <30 mg/dl or >400 mg/dl, ionic calcium <0.8 mEq/l, base deficit >−10.

V. Other patients at risk of organ failure or system failure.

VI. Toxic exposed patients in which none of the above are present but:

- Within a few hours, one of the above criteria is expected.
- Suicide patient that cannot be monitored in other unit care.

## 3. Specific monitoring and treatment in PICU

The main concern in the management of a patient with acute intoxication in PICU is the support of the vital functions. The general measures in a poisoned patient do not differ significantly from those required in a patient admitted to PICU with similar symptoms and a comparable level of severity but with pathology [4]. These critically intoxicated patients should be rapidly recognized by the clinician and evaluated for appropriate therapy. Continuous follow-up of vital functions, neurological status, blood volume, and heart rate makes possible early detection of poisoning worsening signs requiring rapid intervention to prevent complications [5]. Advanced medical technology in PICU offers a number of invasive and noninvasive options that can trigger an early warning of rapid deterioration or provide feedback about the response to treatment. For example, monitoring hemodynamic parameters are valuable for managing poisoned patients with hypotension, volume depletion, or respiratory failure from acute lung injury (ALI). Most importantly, clinicians need to recognize that no monitoring device improves clinical outcome unless is completed by a treatment.

Some antidotes and specific therapies are initiated in ED and continued in PICU, which is the most appropriate place to administer or continue treatment. In addition to conventional therapies, PICU's medical practitioners also know how to deal with situations that do not look like treatment protocols. For example, high doses of atropine, like hundreds of milligrams, can be used to treat organophosphate insecticides [5, 10]. Sometimes the antidote has less effect than the toxin. For example, opioid-intoxicated coma patients responding to naloxone are rapidly recovering. But these patients should be closely monitored for rejoining their coma, and in this situation, the antidote should be repeated. A surveillance period of at least 2 h after the last dose of naloxone is required to assert that the risk of recurrence of toxicity has passed [11].

Pulse oximetry is the recommended method to detect the presence of hypoxemia and to guide the administration of oxygen. Gasometry is a more accurate method for highlighting hypoxemia [4].

## 4. The poisoning effects on specific organ systems

### 4.1 Acute respiratory failure

Acute respiratory failure is a common condition for children with various intoxications to come into the PICU. Respiratory failure occurs due to central hypoventilation, central nervous system depression, by the poisoning of central nervous system depressants (barbiturates, opiates, alcohol, and tranquilizers), intoxication with organophosphate compounds, alkaloids, and atropine. Respiratory muscular paralysis is another mechanism encountered in hemlock poisoning (*Conium maculatum*) and organophosphate. Mechanical ventilation disorders may occur during toxic seizures [12, 13]. Airway obstruction through laryngeal edema is another mechanism of acute respiratory failure encountered in poisoning with corrosive or toxic acidic and toxic bases that cause anaphylactic shock, and obstruction through hypersecretion may occur in intoxication with sympathomimetic substances or organophosphate compounds. Acute toxic respiratory failure may also occur with acute pulmonary edema in alpha-naphthylthiourea (ANTU) intoxications, organophosphate compounds, chlorine, carbon monoxide, ammonia, or hydrogen sulfide. Decreasing oxygenation capacity is another mechanism that can be produced by hemolysis in poisoning with saponin-containing plants or by methemoglobinemia or carboxyhemoglobinemia in nitrite/nitrate intoxication and carbon monoxide intoxication, respectively. The last mechanism consists in altering the oxidative tissue metabolism by inhibiting oxidative systems (cytochromes, cytochromoxidase) that may occur in cyanide, hydrogen sulfide, opaque, or fluorine intoxications [14].

As for the diagnosis of acute toxic respiratory insufficiency, in the initial phase, the signs and symptoms of background intoxication are highlighted. Once the respiratory failure has occurred, its symptoms, which are generally circumscribed to the pathophysiological mechanisms involved, become evident. In acute respiratory failure (ARF) from CNS disorders, consciousness status can be abolished and respiratory movements diminished in amplitude and frequency. The symptoms of ARF by affecting the resilient muscles are dominated by generalized muscular asthenia and dyspnea, and in the ARF by pulmonary damage, the tachypnea is more common. The clinical signs associated with hypercapnia and hypoxia in comatose patients are psychomotor agitation, dyspnea, and cyanosis [4]. However, the severity of cyanosis does not adequately reflect the severity of respiratory insufficiency. Increased intracranial pressure due to cerebral vasodilatation may result in cerebral edema, causing headache, obtundation, and even coma.

Blood gas analysis may reveal respiratory acidosis (pH $< 7.35$ and $PaCO_2 > 45$ mmHg), which can be partially compensated by lowering the alkaline reserve and, in the absence of oxygen therapy, decreasing $PaCO_2$. A serious form of acute respiratory failure is acute respiratory distress syndrome (ARDS) manifested by bilateral pulmonary infiltration on radiography, $PaO_2/FiO_2$ ratio (partial oxygen pressure in arterial blood/oxygen fraction in the inspired air) below 200 mmHg and hemodynamic parameters within normal limits [12].

Corticosteroids and antibiotics may be used for the prophylactic purposes. Corticosteroids have been used for many toxic inhalational injuries. The prophylactic treatment of patients with inhalation injury with antibiotics has a empirical support [14, 15]. Essential therapy aims to ensure adequate blood oxygenation. Ensuring the ventilatory support should be seen in dynamics. Thus, ventilatory support begins with the least invasive supportive methods and progresses to the most aggressive techniques; you must minimize risks such as pneumothorax [16]. Oxygen supplementation is indicated for patients with suspected or confirmed respiratory failure.

Approximately 10% of children admitted to the PICU for poisoning may require endotracheal intubation [6]. After the decision for mechanical ventilation has been made, the route needs to be selected. Some experts prefer oral intubation because it allows the use of a larger endotracheal tube—usually 8 mm or more in adults—than nasal intubation [17]. A wide range of equipment is necessary to allow for a wide range of patient size. A selection of both straight and curved blades should be available. Capnography should be available to assist the endotracheal tube placement in the airway.

The goal of mechanical ventilation is to provide a sufficient exchange of oxygen and carbon dioxide and the metabolic needs of a patient to be accomplished with minimum adverse effects [4]. The purpose of mechanical ventilation is not always to achieve the normal blood gas concentration. Given the predisposition to hypoventilation and the risk of acute pulmonary edema, the mechanical ventilation of patients intoxicated with salicylates requires a lot of attention [18, 19]. High-frequency ventilation and ECMO should be considered to treat some severe intoxications, but there are limited reports on their use in pediatric toxicology [4, 20].

Noninvasive ventilation refers to providing the ventilation support without an invasive artificial path (intubation or tracheostomy probe). Patient selection is made taking into account noninvasive ventilation indications and contraindications as well as predictive factors of success or failure. Before starting noninvasive ventilation, a plan should be established to be applied if therapy fails. Noninvasive ventilation can be done with either portable CPAP or BiPAP devices that can also be used for home ventilation with either intensive ventilation or portable ventilation. One of the common causes of failure of noninvasive ventilation is the large air loss around to the ventilation mask [21].

### 4.2 Neurological complications

These are often the most prevalent symptoms in accidental or voluntary poisonings. Acute voluntary poisonings often involve psychotropic drugs (anxiolytic-hypnotic, antidepressant, antipsychotic, etc.) or ethanol, whose central toxic target is the central nervous system. If the alteration of consciousness is a frequent complication of poisoning, mortality directly attributable to neurological impairment is small compared to other etiologies (traumatic, vascular, etc.). Alteration of consciousness is most often due to a functional and reversible nature. It results from an interaction with one or more essential neurotransmitters (gamma-acidobutyric acid, serotonin, dopamine, etc.). However, lesional damage remains possible in case of exposure to a toxicant that prevents oxygen cellular use (e.g., carbon monoxide), when late detection or cardiopulmonary resuscitation complications cause anoxic or ischemic brain injury and ultimately neurovascular lesions [4, 22].

#### *4.2.1 Acute alteration of consciousness*

This is one of the most common pediatric emergencies. Its most serious form, coma, is one of the most critical situations faced by a doctor. Child coma occurs on an immature and fragile brain. In all cases of coma under the age of 7 years (including accidental poisoning), there is a risk that child's natural development achievements process will be compromised because the damage to the nervous system occurs during the full development process [23, 24]. The central nervous system (CNS), due to its rich lipid content and abundant vascularization is frequently the target organ for many toxic and nontoxic drugs. In intoxications, coma may occur due to direct toxic effects, metabolic abnormalities, or toxic-induced anoxia [25, 26].

The frequency of toxic coma varies in different studies, from 5% [26] to 28.9% [27]. In a recent prospective observational study, they accounted for 11.5% of all nontraumatic coma [28].

##### *4.2.1.1 Anamnestic and clinical diagnosis of toxic comas*

The toxic etiology of a coma must be raised in any patient who presents a severe deterioration of consciousness, without another obvious cause. In the absence of seizures, the patient often progresses to coma passing through the stages of lethargy, confusion, and stupor. A carefully conducted anamnesis, taken from the caregivers, can sometimes indicate a poisoning. The child's age can provide important information. Small children are prone to accidental poisoning, and in this situation, questioning the caregivers about toxic substances found in the house may be useful. Adolescents tend to experience alcohol, psychoactive substances, or recreational drugs. In the absence of an obvious history, toxicological exams need to be conducted in serum and urine [29, 30].

The physical examination can also provide clues about a possible intoxication. Thus, a careful examination of the teguments may reveal signs of venous punctures suggesting a drug self-injection, including heroin. Sclero-tegumentary jaundice may be highlighted, suggesting a hepatic failure of a toxic cause that has evolved into a coma. Epistaxis may exist in snorting cocaine. The presence of head lesions should alert the doctor about the possibility of a possible simultaneous cranial trauma [31]. The vital signs are also important for orientation toward a toxic etiology. For example, benzodiazepines and opiates often cause respiratory depression. Amphetamines and cocaine can cause hypertension and tachyarrhythmias. Drugs that affect the autonomic nervous system may induce hyperthermia, vasoconstriction or vasodilatation, and heart rhythm disorders [32].

Neurological examination is very important for the diagnosis (**Figure 1**). Evaluation of the coma is important in unconscious patients (**Table 1**). The general characteristics of toxic coma are the absence of meningeal signs and neurological focal signs, unless hypoglycemia is involved. During neurological examination, the plantar, deep tendon reflex, and muscle tone must be examined. Depending on the changes found, one of the following three syndromes can be outlined: pyramidal, extrapyramidal, or myorelaxation, which may indicate the toxins involved in inducing coma.

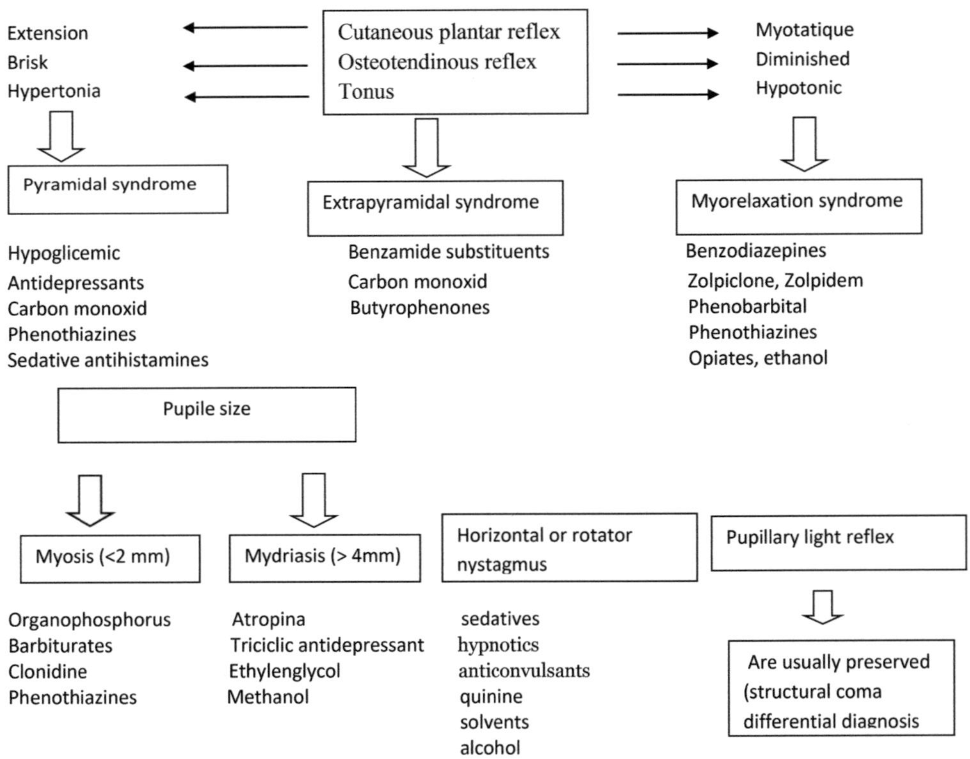


**Figure 1.**
*Neurological examination of the patient with toxic coma [33].*

| Area assessed | Infant | Children | Score |
|---|---|---|---|
| Eyeopening | Open spontaneously | Open spontaneously | 4 |
| | Open in response to verbal stimuli | Open in response to verbal stimuli | 3 |
| | Open in response to pain only | Open in response to pain only | 2 |
| | No response | No response | 1 |
| Verbalresponse | Coos and babbles | Oriented, appropriate | 5 |
| | Verbal response | Confused | 4 |
| | Cries in response to pain | Inappropriate words | 3 |
| | Moans in response to pain | Incomprehensible words or nonspecific sounds | 2 |
| | No response | No response | 1 |
| Motor response | Moves spontaneously and purposefully | Obeys commands | 6 |
| | Withdraws to touch | Localizes painful stimulus | 5 |
| | Withdraws in response to pain | Withdraws in response to pain | 4 |
| | Responds to pain with decorticate posturing (abnormal flexion) | Responds to pain with decorticate posturing (abnormal flexion) | 3 |
| | Responds to pain with decerebrate posturing (abnormal extension) | Responds to pain with decerebrate posturing (abnormal extension) | 2 |
| | No response | No response | 1 |

**Table 1.**
*Modified Glasgow coma scale for infants and children.*

Eye exams are essential for the toxic etiology. The type of coma associated with pupillary response may also suggest the toxin responsible for the coma appearance [33–35] (**Figure 1**). Periodic movement type "ping-pong" has been described in poisoning with monoamine oxidase inhibitors [34]. Hyperthermia is part of the anticholinergic syndrome; when associated with neurological disorders and toxic ingestion is not evident, then it is necessary to search for a *cerebromeningeal* infectious cause [31]. A convulsive coma may occur in the evolution of a poisoning with tricyclic antidepressants, phenothiazines, antihistamines, lithium, theophylline, carbamazepine, dextropropoxyphene, amphetamines, cocaine, and hypoglycemic substances [35]. Coma associated with hemodynamic disorders can be found in meprobamate poisoning, membrane stabilizers, calcium inhibitors, or beta-blockers [4]. Detecting some breathing disorders associated with coma may be suggestive of some toxics. Decreased respiratory rate below 12 breaths/min, with regular breathing, indicates opioids or sedative hypnotics. Some sympathomimetic agents (salicylates, amphetamines, CO) on the contrary stimulate breathing, causing tachypnea. Kussmaul-type breathing (high frequency, regular) is usually associated with metabolic acidosis from poisonings with ethylene glycol, methanol, or salicylates [36, 37].

#### *4.2.1.2 Laboratory investigations*

Useful investigations into a toxic coma are mainly in serum determinations and much less often in neuroimaging investigations. Any metabolic acidosis in a toxic coma requires further investigation. The presence of low anionic gap suggests lithium or bromine intoxication. Highlighting an osmolar gap usually indicates a poisoning with ethanol, isopropanol, methanol, or ethylene glycol. Pure respiratory acidosis is consistent with hypoventilation, possibly a sign of poisoning with hypnotic sedatives or opioids. Although urinary toxicological tests may sometimes be useful in a toxic coma, the results are often false positive or false negative [24, 25].

Dosage of serum concentrations of some drugs is of great help, if available. Other useful investigations are the dosage of serum cholinesterases and carboxyhemoglobin. Coma caused by tricyclic antidepressants poisoning may be accompanied by electrocardiographic abnormalities (dysrhythmia) and seizures [38].

*4.2.1.3 Treatment*

The main life threat in toxic coma is the alteration of respiratory function. Therefore, maintaining airway permeability and ensuring effective breathing are a priority, because providing the $O_2$ requirement of the brain is essential. In any suspicion of hypoxia or CO intoxication, $O_2$ should be administered [32]. Not every child in a toxic coma should be intubated. It is estimated that orotracheal intubation is required in about 20% of toxic coma. The main indications are coma with alteration of swallow reflexes, acute respiratory failure unresponsive to $O_2$ administration, severe circulatory insufficiency or toxic comas associated with severe symptoms, refractory to pharmacological treatment (convulsions, hyperthermia) [33].

Glycemia should be measured as a matter of urgency, and if there is hypoglycemia, this must be quickly rectified. Activated charcoal gastrointestinal decontamination can sometimes provide benefits, if done early. Gastric lavage can be performed if the patient has the respiratory tract protected by endotracheal tube. If the toxic is adsorbed on the activated charcoal, it can be administered by nasogastric tube. There is a lot of attention needed when administered to non-intubated patients. Hemodynamic instability induced by toxic shock, which may be hypovolemic, distributive, or cardiogenic, requires vascular filling with saline or Ringer's solution, injected quickly and possibly vasopressor medication. Any detected heart rhythm disorders and hypertension or hypotension need to be corrected. Simultaneously with the stabilization measures, the antidote will be administered according to the protocols in toxic-induced coma [25].

In comas of unknown etiology, the concept of "coma cocktail" containing dextrose, oxygen, naloxone, and thiamine (vitamin B1) was proposed. But indications and efficiency were controversial.

Currently, in toxic comas, precise indications for flumazenil and naloxone are used. Flumazenil acts by a competitive mechanism at the benzodiazepine receptor level, canceling the sedation effects of benzodiazepines within 1–2 min of administration. In the case of children, we start with a dose of 0.01 mg/kg intravenously, which can be repeated 1–2 min to a total dose of 0.05 mg/kg maximum 1 mg. It is effective in toxic-induced coma by zolpidem and zopiclone. If in a calm coma of undetermined etiology, there is no patient awakening after the administration of flumazenil referred to dose, the diagnosis of intoxication with benzodiazepines is infirmed [39]. Naloxone is a pure opioid antagonist, which acts by competitive antagonism at μ receptors to determine the reversibility of respiratory depression, hypotension, and miotic within 2 min. For children >3 years, the indicated dose is 0.01–0.1 mg/kg. If the desired effect is obtained, it may be repeated two times at an interval of 5 min; the dose may reach 10 mg. Regardless of the way of administration (intravenous, subcutaneous, intramuscular, endotracheal intubation probe, or inhalation), the effect is similar. The lack of response within 15 min after administration requires looking for another coma cause [4, 5].

Extrarenal epuration may sometimes have indications in coma due to alcohol intoxications (ethylene glycol, isopropyl alcohol, and methanol), salicylates, theophylline, lithium, valproic acid, carbamazepine, or carbamates [40].

#### *4.2.1.4 Prognosis*

The prognosis of toxic coma is generally better than that of anoxic coma. For example, in sedative poisoning, mortality is below 1%. The following neurological signs provide a poor prognosis for recovery from toxic coma: absence of corneal reflexes after day 1, absence of eye opening response on day 3, loss of pupillary reflexes (up to 1 week), lack of oculovestibular response, abnormal skeletal muscle tonus, the absence of spontaneous eye movement, the isoelectric pathway on the electroencephalogram [25].

Some toxic may cause prolonged coma (>100 h) with intermittent agitation periods known as cyclic coma: barbiturates, carbamazepine, clonazepam, ethchlorvynol, glutethimide, meprobamate, olanzapine, quetiapine. Short-term memory alteration and postcoma amnesia are possible, secondary to neuron damage in the pyramidal system at the hippocampus level in CO intoxication [25, 38].

### *4.2.2. Convulsions*

Convulsions are common in situations when the toxic involved affects the central nervous system. In the context of poisoning, seizures are often a sign of severity [41]. From the clinical point of view, toxic-induced convulsions can occur with or without warning signs (e.g., aura) or mental state alteration. Most toxic-induced seizures are generalized, tonic–clonic ("grand mal"). Epileptic status is defined as a continuous convulsive activity lasting more than 30 min or more convulsive episodes between which consciousness is not completely regained [4, 5, 42]. Patients with preexisting epileptogenic focal conditions may experience focal seizures [42].

#### *4.2.2.1 Etiology of toxic seizures*

**Table 2** presents the etiology of toxic seizures.

#### *4.2.2.2 Treatment of toxic seizures*

Seizure control in PICU is a fundamental problem in the management of a poisoned child. Convulsions associated with toxic ingestion are sometimes difficult to control, being recurrent or persistent leading to status epileptics. This is associated with an increase in oxygen in the brain level. The imbalance between supply and demand can lead to cerebral ischemia. That is why an aggressive management of toxic seizures is critical to preventing brain damage. The first priority in managing seizure crises is to provide airway permeability and oxygen therapy to ensure delivery of oxygen to the brain. Evaluation and correction of electrolyte disturbances and hypoglycemia should also be promptly performed [4, 43]. The first therapeutic line for toxic-induced convulsions is represented by benzodiazepines (diazepam, lorazepam, or midazolam). Lorazepam and diazepam exhibit a similar clinical response time (until termination of seizure activity) [41, 42]. However, after treatment with lorazepam, the rate of seizure recurrence appears to be lower [44]. Also, according to some studies, lorazepam has been shown to have a longer duration of action of the anticonvulsant effect (12–24 h vs. 15–30 min) and is therefore the preferred choice of some clinicians [42]. The preferred route of administration of benzodiazepines is intravenous. **Table 3** lists the doses of benzodiazepines that can be used in toxic-induced convulsions in children and adolescents.

In the absence of response to benzodiazepines, phenobarbital or valproic acid may be effective for crises control. Phenytoin is less effective in the treatment of induced seizures [42]. If seizures do not stop at the referred medication, it is

| Class | Example(s) | Class | Example(s) |
|---|---|---|---|
| **Pharmaceuticals** | | **Nonpharmaceuticals** | |
| Analgesics | Meperidine/normeperidine, propoxyphene, pentazocine, salicylate, tramadol | Alcohols | Methanol, ethanol (withdrawal) |
| Anesthetics | Local anesthetics *(lidocaine, benzocaine)* | Antiseptic/ preservatives | Ethylene oxide, phenol |
| Anticonvulsants | Carbamazepine | Biologic toxins | |
| Antidepressants | Tricyclic (amitriptilina/ nortriptyline), amoxapine, bupropion, selective serotonin reuptake inhibitors (citalopram), venlafaxine | Marine animals, mushrooms, plants | Domoic acid [shellfish (blue mussels)], monomethylhydrazine (*Gyromitra* spp.), coniine (poison hemlock), virol A (water hemlock), camphor |
| Antihistamines | Diphenhydramine, doxylamine, tripelennamine | Gases (naturally and/or anthropogenically occurring) | Carbon monoxide, hydrogen sulfide, cyanide |
| Antimicrobials | Antibacterials (selected penicillins, cephalosporins, carbapenems, fluoroquinolones), antimalarials (chloroquine), tuberculostatics (isoniazid) | Metals/ organometallics | Alkyl mercurials (dimethylmercury), arsenic, lead, thallium, tetraethyl lead, organotins (trimethyltin) |
| Antineoplastics | Alkylating agents (busulfan, chlorambucil) | Metal hydrides | Pentaborane, phosphine |
| Antipsychotics | Clozapine, loxapine | Pesticides | |
| Antiasthmatic | Theophylline | Fungicides/ herbicides | Dinitrophenol, diquat, glufosinate |
| Cardiovascular drug | Propranolol, quinidine | Insecticides | Organochlorines (DDT, lindane), organophosphates (parathion), pyrethroids (type II), sulfuryl fluoride, alkylhalides (methyl bromide) |
| Cholinergics | Pilocarpine, bethanechol | Molluscicides | Metaldehyde |
| Muscle relaxants | Baclofen, orphenadrine | Rodenticides | Strychnine, zinc, or aluminum phosphide |
| Nonsteroidal anti-inflammatory drug | Mefenamic acid, phenylbutazone | | |
| Psychostimulant/ anorectics | Amphetamine, caffeine, cocaine, methamphetamine, 3,4-methylenedioxymethamphetamine, synthetic cannabinoids | | |
| Vitamins/ supplements | Vitamin A, ferrous sulfate | | |

**Table 2.**
*Proconvulsant agents (adapted after Hanson [44]).*

necessary to induce coma with sodium thiopental or propofol. To induce a coma, sodium thiopental is administered as a bolus of 3 mg/kg, which is repeated after 2 min, followed by maintenance with 1–15 mg/kg/h. For propofol, the dose is 1–5 mg/kg bolus (repeatable) followed by continuous infusion up to a maximum

| Benzodiazepine | Pediatric dose |
|---|---|
| Lorazepam | 0.05–0.1 mg/kg iv (maximum 4 mg/dose). It can be repeated at 10–15 min if necessary. Maximum dose: 8 mg/12 h |
| Diazepam | <5 years: 0.2–0.5 mg/kg iv every 2–5 min up to a maximum total dose of 5 mg.<br>>5 years: 1–2 mg iv every 2–5 min up to a maximum total dose of 10 mg. |
| Midazolam | >2 months: 0.15 mg/kg iv bolus, followed by a continuous infusion of 1 μg/kg/min, titrating the dose every 5 min until seizure control. Mean dose: 2–3 μg/kg/min. |

**Table 3.**
*Posology of benzodiazepines in seizures in childhood (adapted after Blais and Dubé [41]).*

of 5 mg/kg/h [45]. A special category of seizure, which does not respond to traditional therapy, is that of isoniazid intoxication. In this case, the crises result from exhaustion of pyridoxine (vitamin B6) and respond only to its administration [4]. In case of intoxication with isoniazid, the vitamin B6 posology is 1 gram per gram of ingested isoniazid (maximum 5 grams). This dose will be given slowly within 10 min, or until seizures cease. If the seizures stop during administration, the remaining dose will be given within the next 4 h. If the dose of isoniazid is unknown, 70 mg/kg iv (maximum 5 g) should be administered in the same manner. The initial dose may be repeated once seizures relapse. Pyridoxine is also anticonvulsant therapy of choice in intoxication with gyromitra mushrooms in the dose of 25 mg/kg iv in 10 min and can be repeated in case of seizure recurrence [41].

### 4.3 Cardiovascular disorders

These are a serious complication of some poisoning, requiring prompt monitoring and treatment. Assessing a poisoned child at risk of cardiovascular disease requires a detailed physical exam. In addition to cardiac volume and output evaluation, a series of laboratory tests must be performed: blood gases, electrolyte dosing, blood sugar, transaminases, and azote retention tests. In some cases, the serum level of the toxic substance can also be determined, which helps to assess the severity of intoxication and to support the therapeutic decision. Additional care management such as blood pressure measurement, electrocardiography, and echocardiography can also be useful to guide therapy in case of a poisoning accompanied by cardiovascular instability. Identification of a certain toxic can simplify the treatment through specific intervention. If the poison is unknown, the initial resuscitation consists in administration of intravenous fluids to maintain a proper intravascular volume [4, 5]. Rapid administration of 20 ml/kg bolus isotonic fluids, usually crystalloid (normal saline or Ringer's lactate) over 10–15 min, is used to restore intravascular volume. Additional fluid bolus may be required depending on the reassessment of intravascular volume [46]. However, the intravascular volume should be corrected cautiously, because too vigorous expansion may lead to fluid retention, liver enlargement, signs of pulmonary edema, jugular vein distension, or cardiomegaly, without improvement of vital signs and tissue perfusion. Positively inotropic agents are required in such patients. The cardiovascular disorders, which are present at the time, determine which inotropic agents and vasopressor drugs to choose.

Arrhythmia is a frequent complication in cardiovascular drug poisoning. Dysrhythmia may occur by direct affecting of the electrical conduction system of the heart, by changing the electrical membrane potential across the myocardial cell, or by indirect disturbance of the electrical conduction system through the nervous system or due to electrolytic and metabolic disorders, which affect the electrical activity of the heart.

### *4.3.1 Bradyarrhythmias: etiology and treatment*

Bradyarrhythmias occur due to some toxic substances, which decrease the central nervous system influx or the chronotropic activity of the conduction system. Agents that can induce bradyarrhythmias are tricyclic antidepressants, α2-adrenergic agonists, β-adrenergic blockers, calcium channel blockers, cholinomimetics, digoxin, sedative hypnotics, organophosphorus and carbamates, plants containing cardiac glycosides, opioids, cocaine, organophosphorus, and carbamates [47].

Bradyarrhythmia due to ingestion of unknown toxic substance is managed with supportive treatment. Atropine or positive inotropic agents, such as epinephrine, are used to correct bradyarrhythmia. When the toxic agent is known, the aim of the therapy is to antagonize the toxic effects (e.g., calcium chloride is used to treat calcium channel blockers intoxication). Literature data showed that in poisoning with β-blocker, calcium channel blocker, and tricyclic antidepressant, glucagon may be used, given its positive inotropic and chronotropic effects. Glucagon dose in children is 0.03–0.15 mg/kg in 1–2 min bolus, followed by 0.07 mg/kg/h infusion or by repeated boluses in 5–10 min, as needed [48]. Other therapies that may be used in severe β-blocker and calcium channel blocker poisoning are hyperinsulinemia—euglycemia (HIE) and intravenous fat emulsion (IFE) [49]. In bradycardia mediated by vagal reflex, atropine is the treatment of choice. For unresponsive sinus bradycardia, as well as for junctional or ventricular bradyarrhythmias, isoproterenol may be used. Specific therapy should also be used (calcium in calcium channel blockers intoxication; digoxin antibodies in digoxin poisoning). Sodium bicarbonate is beneficial in tricyclic antidepressant poisoning. Concomitant correction of electrolyte disturbances, hypoxia, and acidosis is mandatory because they may contribute to failure of pacing stimulus to depolarize cardiac cells [47]. In severe cases of bradyarrhythmia or heart block unresponsive to pharmacological therapy, direct transthoracic pacing may be necessary.

### *4.3.2 Tachyarrhythmias*

Tachyarrhythmias are common in poisonings. They are classified as wide-complex and narrow-complex rhythm (**Tables 4** and 5).

Electrocardiogram (ECG) in narrow-complex tachyarrhythmias shows sinus tachycardia or supraventricular tachycardia (normal conduction).

Specific therapies include antidotes depending on xenobiotic. Treatment imposes corrections of hypotension, hypoxia, or electrolyte abnormalities and administration of esmolol or other short-acting beta-blocker for intractable tachycardia in the absence of hypotension or other signs of myocardial depression [4, 47].

ECG in wide-complex tachyarrhythmias may show ventricular tachycardia (VT) monomorphic or polymorphic, ventricular fibrillation (VF), ECG signs preceding

| |
|---|
| **Anticholinergic:** amantadine, antihistamines, atropine, belladonna, scopolamine, cyclic antidepressants, mushrooms (muscarine-containing, e.g., clitocybe dealbata), neuroleptics (thioridazines and mesoridazines also are membrane depressants), plants (e.g., Jimson weed) |
| **Sympathomimetic:** amphetamines and their congeners (e.g., ecstasy), caffeine, chloral hydrate, cocaine, ethanol, ephedrine and pseudoephedrine, lysergic acid diethylamide (LSD) and other hallucinogens, monoamine oxidase inhibitors, phencyclidine, scorpion or spider envenomation, sedative-hypnotic withdrawal, selective serotonin reuptake inhibitors, theophylline |
| **Cholinomimetic:** organophosphates |

**Table 4.**
*Poisoning-induced narrow-complex tachyarrhythmias.*

| |
|---|
| Antiarrhythmics (type Ia, Ic, III), antihistamines, arsenic, cardiac glycosides, cyclic antidepressants, carbamazepine, chloral hydrate |
| **Other toxic**: sodium fluoride, freon (and other fluorocarbon aerosols), hydrocarbon solvents, neuroleptics, propoxyphene, quinine, and related agents |

**Table 5.**
*Poisoning-induced wide-complex tachyarrhythmias.*

VF/VT, supraventricular tachyarrhythmias, prominent R wave lead AVR, rightward deviation of QRS axis, and QT prolongation [47].

Correction of possible hydroelectrolytic and acido-basic imbalance is required in treatment of toxic ventricular tachycardia. In monomorphic ventricular tachycardia, if the patient's condition is stable and there is no hemodynamic instability, chemical cardioversion with amiodarone 5 mg/kg iv, or procainamide 15 mg/kg iv or lidocaine 1 mg/kg bolus is first attempted. In wide QRS complex tachycardias, adenosine is not useful. If the chemical cardioversion has results, the drug will be administered by continuous intravenous infusion to avoid relapses. The IV infusion time will be decided along with the pediatric cardiologist. If the chemical cardioversion is ineffective, synchronized biphasic electrical cardioversion with 0.5–1 J/kg is needed [47, 50]. In polymorphic ventricular tachycardia with hemodynamic instability, the treatment is based on electrical cardioversion associated with magnesium. If magnesium sulfate is ineffective or bradyarrhythmias occur, isoproterenol IV may be useful. Hypokalemia can exacerbate ventricular tachycardia, and therefore, potassium supplementation is required even in patients with normal potassium at the time of determination.

Bidirectional ventricular tachycardia is a hallmark of severe digitalis toxicity, and immediate specific antidote treatment with FAB antibodies must be started. This type of ventricular tachycardia may occur in aconite poisoning too [51, 52].

Torsades de pointes (TdP) is a specific type of polymorphic ventricular tachycardia exhibiting a characteristic morphology on the electrocardiogram, in which the QRS complexes "twist" around the isoelectric line. This is a major toxin-induced arrhythmia, which may degenerate into ventricular fibrillation and sudden death [53, 54]. In this situation, the corrections of electrolyte disorders, bradycardia, acidosis, low blood pressure, and hypoxia are needed. If poisoning involves a drug with $Na^+$ channel blocking properties (e.g., tricyclic antiarrhythmic drugs, cocaine, class IA and IC antiarrhythmic drugs, or antipsychotic drugs), sodium bicarbonate may be used to reduce the degree of sodium channel blockade by increasing extracellular sodium [55]. The treatment of choice in torsade de pointes is magnesium sulfate. The pediatric dose is 25–50 mg/kg iv. If a poisoned patient does not respond to the abovementioned therapeutic measures, intravenous lipid emulsion therapy should be considered if the drug has lipophilic properties. A last therapeutic alternative is arteriovenous extracorporeal membrane oxygenation (ECMO) [47, 55].

## 5. Techniques for extrarenal treatment in toxicology

The Extracorporeal Treatments in Poisoning (EXTRIP) Workgroup is a group of international experts spanning disciplines of nephrology, toxicology, pediatrics, emergency medicine, critical care, and clinical pharmacologists that has been reviewing the evidence in the literature and provide recommendations for the use of extracorporeal treatments in poisonings. To date, EXTRIP has published systematic reviews on the role of extracorporeal treatment (ECTR) for poisoning from acetaminophen, barbiturates, carbamazepine, digoxin, lithium, metformin, methanol, salicylates, thallium, theophylline, tricyclic antidepressants, and valproic acid [56]. Waste treatment methods are numerous, and techniques and/or equipment continuously evolve. It mainly involves hemodialysis, hemoperfusion, hemofiltration, and albumin dialysis [57].

## 5.1 Hemodialysis

Hemodialysis is the technique of removing toxins from the blood using a diffusion gradient through a semipermeable membrane. To be dialyzable, poisons must meet the following conditions: hydrosolubility, low molecular weight, apparent low volume of distribution, low protein binding, and low endogenous clearance [5]. It may be necessary in the following situations: severe poisoning with salicylates, accompanied by important mental disorders, in some phenobarbital intoxications, ethylene glycol, lithium, and theophylline [4, 6].

Possible complications of hemodialysis are hypotension, hypoxemia, bleeding, embolism, and cardiac rhythm disorders [4].

## 5.2 Hemoperfusion

The hemoperfusion column can be considered as an extracorporeal clearance organ, increasing the overall clearance of the body. Its efficacy is superior to hemodialysis or hemofiltration. It has been proposed in serious poisonings with theophylline, carbamazepine, and cardiotoxic (membrane stabilizers, inhibitors calculation, and meprobamate) that do not quickly respond well to symptomatic treatment led. Its indication should be taken into account very early and in intoxications with some toxic lesions such as colchicine or paraquat [57]. Complications of hemoperfusion can be thrombocytopenia (30%), leukopenia (10%), hypocalcemia, hypoglycemia, reduction of fibrinogen, and hypothermia. The future lies in hemoperfusion devices coated with drug-specific antibodies or the antidote of the toxin instead of activated charcoal [58].

## 5.3 Hemofiltration and hemodiafiltration

Hemofiltration and hemodiafiltration have similar properties as hemodialysis regarding the distribution volume and protein-binding percentage. Water-like substances move out of the plasma through the membrane, and this fluid is replaced with isotonic fluids. The rate of removal of the toxin is influenced by the degree of protein binding and the ultrafiltration (UF) and the sieving coefficient, which is the ability of the solute to cross a membrane by convection. Although this makes high-efficiency convective techniques suitable for poisoning, reports of their use in poisoned patients remain limited due to their higher technical requirements and lesser availability [58, 59].

## 5.4 Other purification techniques used in toxicology

The most developed and most commonly used hepatic dialysis systems are the molecular adsorbent recirculation (MARS) and fractional plasma separation and absorption (Prometheus).

### *5.4.1 MARS albumin dialysis*

MARS is a hemodialysis technique that combines the selective removal of albumin-bound toxins with the removal of water-soluble toxins. The MARS system uses a 20% human albumin solution as a dialyzate and a semipermeable membrane as a dialyzer.

The albumin acquires an increased ability to bind toxins through contact with membrane's polymers. Through the membrane, the patient's blood comes into contact with the albumin solution, and the albumin-related toxins cross the membrane and enter the dialyzate, the transfer being made in the sense of the existing concentration gradient between the blood compartment and the albumin solution. After detoxification, the albumin solution is recirculated, coming into contact with the patient's blood again [60–62]. Several small randomized controlled trials and case control studies in adults showed significant improvement, both in morbidity and mortality, in patients treated with MARS. However, there are little data on the use of MARS in the children [63].

#### *5.4.2 The Prometheus system*

It consists of a bloodstream where two filters perform a purification of water-soluble toxins and then a fractional separation of plasma, so that cellular components and macromolecules are separated by albumin and by low-molecular-weight solvents. Then, the autologous albumin solution crosses a neutral resin filter, which has an increased affinity for bile acids, aromatic amino acids, and phenols, and also an anion exchange resin filter that removes unconjugated bilirubin [64–66].

These techniques were initially used in hepatology. Subsequently, they were also used for the treatment of acute poisonings with or without liver failure, especially the MARS technique. The aim is to remove albumin-related toxic substances. There are several reports regarding the use of these purification techniques in high liver toxicity mushrooms poisoning as *Amanita phalloides* [60, 62, 64] and also in paracetamol poisoning [56, 60]. These techniques were also used to treat phenytoin, theophylline, and diltiazem poisoning, and for calcium channel blockers poisoning too [57, 67].

#### *5.4.3 Arteriovenous extracorporeal membrane oxygenation (ECMO)*

ECMO is a special technique for maintaining pulmonary and cardiac function through an extracorporeal circulation pump. The purpose of this method is to provide a good oxygenation support and remove the excess of $CO_2$. It is an exceptional therapy proposed for serious poisonings, especially those that are complicated with respiratory distress syndrome or cardiogenic shock refractor on conventional therapy [68]. ECMO is difficult and should only be done in experienced centers as it carries significant risks. It is a method that requires systemic anticoagulation. The main possible complications are bleeding, systemic infection, and thromboembolic accidents [4, 68]. If the ECMO indication has been established, this therapy should be initiated as soon as possible, before irreversible cerebral or visceral anoxic lesions [68, 69].

## 6. Organ donation

Despite the best efforts of the care team, it is not possible to save every child with poisoning. Particularly, in cases where there was significant hypoxic–ischemic central nervous system injury, patient may progress to brain death [70]. Because poisoning is not a sign of organ donation, these patients can be a potential donor source [71]. Toxicological risk assessment should be rigorously conducted in the sense that the transmission of intoxication to the recipient should be avoided. Some toxic substances accumulate in the liver, heart, or lung and could theoretically be released from these grafts after transplantation. These risks, however, should not be exaggerated. They can be diminished by knowledge of kinetics and toxics in target organs. Taking risks is more important for heart or kidney transplantation, organs that are more susceptible to anoxic-ischemic damage [4–6]. Since severe depression of the central nervous system induced by some toxic can mimic brain death, it is important to allow sufficient time, depending on the pharmacology of the toxic substance, until the plasma concentration decreases to an acceptable level. To declare cerebral death, the following are necessary [4, 72, 73]:

- clinical criteria: deep, dormant coma, absence of brain stem reflexes, absence of spontaneous breathing;

- biological criteria:

    - mandatory: flat track on the EEG, apnea test, atropine test;
    - optional: cerebral angiography (stroke), transcranial echo-Doppler, scintigraphy, etc.

The conditions for declaring brain death vary according to the country's legislation. Basically, the patient's examination should be performed by two physicians: neurologist or neurosurgeon and anesthetist. In children, the intervals between examinations must be 24 h for the child aged 2 months to 1 year and at least 12 h over 1 year [74].

## 7. Conclusion

Complications of poisonings during childhood may enforce hospitalization to PICU and may contribute to lowering the survival rate. Supporting vital functions is the main objective of the management of a poisoned patient admitted in PICU.

## Conflict of interest

None.

## Author details

Nicolai Nistor, Otilia Frăsinariu*, Aniela Rugină, Irina Mihaela Ciomaga and Violeta Ştreangă
Grigore T. Popa University of Medicine and Pharmacy, Iaşi, Romania

*Address all correspondence to: otiliafrasinariu@gmail.com

## References

[1] Madden MA. Pediatric toxicology: Emerging trends. Journal of Pediatric Intensive Care. 2015;**4**:103-110. DOI: 10.1055/s-0035-1556753

[2] Ergul AB, Torun YA. Retrospective evaluation of poisonings in a pediatric intensive care unit: 4 years of experience. Journal of Clinical and Analytical Medicine. 2018;**9**(4):278-283. DOI: 10.4328/JCAM.5660

[3] Lee J, Fan NA, Yao TC, Hsia SH, Lee EP, Huang JL, et al. Clinical spectrum of acute poisoning in children admitted to the pediatric emergency department. Pediatrics and Neonatology. 2018:1-9. DOI: 10.1016/j.pedneo.2018.04.001

[4] Joshi P, Ross MP. Intensive care pediatric poisoning cases. In: Brent J, Burkhart K, Dargan P,Hatten B, Megarbane B, Palmer R, White J, editors. Critical Care Toxicology. Diagnosis and Management of the Critically Poisoned Patient. 2nd ed. Switzerland: Springer International Publishing AG; 2017. pp. 205-222

[5] Kirk MA. Use of the intensive care unit. In: Nelson LS, Lewin NA, Howland MA, Hoffman RS, Goldfrank LR, Flomenbaum NE, editors. Goldfrank's Toxicologic Emergencies. New York: McGraw Hill Medical; 2011. pp. 148-154

[6] Even KM, Armsby CC, Bateman ST. Poisonings requiring admission to the pediatric intensive care unit: A 5-year review. Clinical Toxicology (Philadelphia, PA);**52**(5):519-524. DOI: 10.3109/15563650.2014.909601

[7] Mowry JB, Spyker DA, Brooks DE, Zimmerman A, Schauben JL. 2015 Annual Report of the American Association of Poison Control Centers' National Poison Data System (NPDS): 33rd Annual Report. Clinical Toxicology (Philadelphia, PA). 2016;**54**(10): 924-1109. DOI: 10.1080/15563650.2016

[8] Alanazi MQ, Al-Jeriasy MI, Al-Assiri MH, Afesh LY, Alhammad F, Salam M. Hospital Performance Indicators and Their Associated Factors in Acute Child Poisoning at a Single Poison Center, Central Saudi Arabia. Medicine. 2015;**94**(52):e2339. DOI: 10.1097/MD.0000000000002339

[9] El Masry MK, Azab SMS. Inappropriate management and transfer of cases with acute poisoning referred to poisoning treatment center—Ain Shams University—Cairo. Egyptian Journal of Forensic Sciences. 2013;**3**(1). DOI: 10.1016/j.ejfs.2012.12.001

[10] Karakus A, Celik MM, Karcioglu M, et al. Cases of organophosphate poisoning treated with high-dose of atropine in an intensive care unit and the novel treatment approaches. Toxicology and Industrial Health. 2014;**30**:421-425. DOI: 10.1177/0748233712462478

[11] Beheshti A, Lucas L, Dunz T, Haydash M, Chiodi H, Edmiston B, et al. An evaluation of naloxone use for opioid overdoses in West Virginia: A literature review. American Medical Journal. 2015;**6**(1):9-13. DOI: 10.3844/amjsp.2015.9.13

[12] McKay CA. Toxin-induced respiratory distress. Emergency Medicine Clinics of North America. 2014;**32**(1):127-147. DOI: 10.1016/j.emc.2013.09.003

[13] Gorguner M, Akgun M. Acute inhalation injury. Eurasian Journal of Medicine. 2010;**42**:28-35. DOI: 10.5152/eajm.2010.09

[14] de Lange DW. Treatment of acute respiratory distress syndrome in the poisoned patient. In: Brent J, Burkhart K, Dargan P,Hatten B, Megarbane B, Palmer R, White J, editors. Critical Care Toxicology. Diagnosis and Management

of the Critically Poisoned Patient. 2nd ed. Switzerland: Springer International Publishing AG; 2017. pp. 359-384

[15] Anan K, Ichikado K, Kawamura K, Johkoh T, Fujimoto K, Suga M. Clinical characteristics and prognosis of drug-associated acute respiratory distress syndrome compared with nondrug-associated acute respiratory distress syndrome: A single-Centre retrospective study in Japan. BMJ Open. 2017;7:e015330. DOI: 10.1136/bmjopen-2016-015330

[16] da Silva PSL, de Aguiar VE, Fonseca MCM. Iatrogenic pneumothorax in mechanically ventilated children: Incidence, risk factors and other outcomes. Journal of Acute and Critical Care. 2015;**44**(3):238-242. DOI: 10.1016/j.hrtlng.2015.01.005

[17] Stolbach A, Hoffman RS. Respiratory principle. In: Nelson LS, Lewin NA, Howland MA, Hoffman RS, Goldfrank LR, Flomenbaum NE, editors. Goldfrank's Toxicologic Emergencies. New York: McGraw Hill Medical; 2011. pp. 303-313

[18] Santo RE, Vaz S, Jalles F, Boto L, Abecasis F. Salicylate intoxication in an infant: A case report. Drug Safety—Case Reports. 2017;**4**:22-25

[19] Shively RM, Hoffman RS, Manini AF. Acute salicylate poisoning: Risk factors for severe outcome. Clinical Toxicology (Philadelphia, PA). 2017;**55**(3):175-180. DOI: 10.1080/15563650.2016.1271127

[20] Moniz M, Silvestre C, Nunes P, et al. High-frequency oscillatory ventilation in children: A 10-year experience. Jornal de Pediatria. 2013;**89**:48-55. DOI: 10.1016/j.jped.2013.02.008

[21] André-von Arnim AO, Jamal SM, John-Stewart GC, Musa NL, Roberts J, Stanberry LI, et al. Pediatric respiratory support technology and practices: A global survey. Healthcare. 2017;**5**(34): 1-11. DOI: 10.3390/healthcare5030034

[22] Monat-Descamps C, Deschamps F. Nervous system disorders induced by occupational and environmental toxic exposure. Open Journal of Preventive Medicine. 2012;**2**(3):272-278. DOI: 10.4236/ojpm.2012.23039

[23] Brissaud O. Coma nontraumatique chez l'enfant. 16emes Journées d'Urgences Pédiatriques de Sud Ouest 2015. http://www.jupso.fr/file/medtool/webmedtool/hodetool01/botm0072/pdf00001.pdf?fbclid=IwAR3y_3RZCuZFLZjQwfduwgcNlFVxXOMc2b3uRJp2wMSMiJ7YvSzhLloJr7g

[24] Oriot D. Coma. In: Labrune P, Oriot D, Labrune B, Huault G, editors. Urgences pédiatriques du prematuré a l'adolescent. Paris: De Boeck et Estem; 2010. pp. 635-645

[25] Leikin JB,Carlson A. Toxicant-induced alteration in consciousness. In: Brent J, Burkhart K, Dargan P,Hatten B, Megarbane B, Palmer R, White J, editors. Critical Care Toxicology. Diagnosis and Management of the Critically Poisoned Patient. 2nd ed. Springer; 2017. pp. 425-446

[26] Sarin SM, Debabrata G, Marami D. Study of etiological profile and outcome predictors in nontraumatic coma. International Journal of Medical Research & Health Sciences. 2016;**5**(6):122-126

[27] Owolabi LF, Mohammed AD, Dalhat MM, Ibrahim A, Aliyu S, Owolabi DS. Factors associated with death and predictors of 1-month mortality in nontraumatic coma in a tertiary hospital in Northwestern Nigeria. Indian Journal of Critical Care Medicine. 2013;**17**(4):219-223. DOI: 10.4103/0972-5229.118422

[28] Ahmad J, Ahmed K, Gattoo IA, Mir MY, Maqbool M, Baba AR. Non traumatic coma in children: A

prospective observational study. International Journal of Contemporary Pediatrics. 2015;**2**(2):77-84. DOI: 10.5455/2349-3291.ijcp20150504

[29] Sachs P, Michot C, Naudin J, Mandre C, Aizenfiza A, Danger S. Coma du nourrisson et de l'enfant: Prise en charge initiale. Réanimation. 2011;**20**:408-418. DOI: 10.1007/s13546-011-0291-6

[30] Suganthi V, Kumar MS, Kumar BRS. Non-traumatic coma in children: A clinical profile and outcome. Journal of Evolution of Medical and Dental Sciences. 2016;**5**(17):867-870. DOI: 10.14260/jemds/2016/200

[31] Claudet I. Quand penser à une intoxication chez l'enfant? Urgences. 2012. https://sofia.medicalistes.fr/spip/IMG/pdf/Quand_penser_a_une_intoxication_chez_l_enfant.pdf

[32] Hantson P. Conduite à tenir devant les encéphalopathies et les comas toxiques. In: Baud F, Hantson P, Thabet H, editors. Intoxications Aiguës. Switzerland: Springer International Publishing AG; 2013. pp. 47-64

[33] Mégarbane B, Donetti L, Blanc T, Chérond G, Jacobse F. Groupe d'experts de la SRLF. Intoxications graves par médicaments et substances illicites en reanimation. Réanimation. 2006;**15**: 332-342

[34] Stancu S, Petran M, Ulmeanu C, Nițescu V. Toxic coma in children etiology and clinical diagnosis. Therapeutics, Pharmacology and Clinical Toxicology. 2011;**15**(1):51-55

[35] Nice P. Le screening toxicologique aux urgences. Congres Urgences. 2010:133-145

[36] Ulmeanu C. Managementul comelor toxice la copil. In: Ulmeanu C, Viorela N, editors. Intoxicațiile acute la copil și adolescent. Oltenita: Tridona; 2015. pp. 68-78

[37] Borgialli DA, Mahajan P, Hoyle JD, Powel EL, Nadet FM, Tunik MG, et al. Performance of the pediatric glasgow coma scale score in the evaluation of children with blunt head trauma. Academic Emergency Medicine. 2016;**23**(8):878-884

[38] De Paepe P, Lemoyne S, Buylaet W. Disorders of consciousness induced by intoxication. Neurologic Clinics. 2012;**30**:359-384. DOI: 10.1016/j.ncl.2011.10.003

[39] Siviloti MLA. Flumazenil, naloxone and the "coma cocktail". British Journal of Clinical Pharmacology. 2015;**81**(3):428-436. DOI: 10.1111/bcp.12731

[40] Bauchman TE, Ferris ME. Management of toxic ingestion with the use of renal replacement therapy. Pediatric Nephrology. 2011;**26**(4):535-541. DOI: 10.1007/s00467-010-1654-3

[41] Blais R, Dubé PA. Traitement des convulsions d'origine toxique. Bulletin d'information toxicologique. 2012;**28**(1):14-19

[42] Chamberlain JM, Okada P, Holsti M, Majan P, Brown KM, Vanc C, et al. Lorazepam vs diazepam for pediatric status epilepticus.a randomized clinical trial. Journal of the American Medical Association. 2014;**311**(16):1652-1660. DOI: 10.1001/jama.2014.2625

[43] Finkelstein Y, Hutson R, Freedman SB, Wax P, Brent J. Drug-induced seizures in children and adolescents presenting for emergency care: Current and emerging trends. Clinical Toxicology. 2013;**51**:761-766

[44] Hanson PF. Toxicant-induced seizures. In: Brent J, Burkhart K, Dargan P, Hatten B, Megarbane B, Palmer R, White J, editors. Critical Care Toxicology. Diagnosis and Management of the Critically Poisoned

Patient. 2nd ed. Switzerland: Springer International Publishing AG; 2017. pp. 447-474

[45] Capovilla G, Beccaria F, Beghi E, Minicucci F, Sartori S, Vecchi M. Treatment of convulsive status epilepticus in childhood: Recommendations of the Italian league against epilepsy. Epilepsia. 2013;**54**(Suppl.7):23-34. DOI: 10.1111/epi.12307

[46] Greenbaum LA. Electrolyte and acid-base disorders. In: Kliegman RM, Stanton BF, Geme JW, Schor NF, editors. Nelson Textbook of Pediatrics. 20th ed. Philadelphia, PA: Elsevier/Saunders; 2016. pp. 346-383

[47] Gugelmann H, Benowitz N. Cardiac conduction and rate disturbances. In: Brent J, Burkhart K, Dargan P, Hatten B, Megarbane B, Palmer R, White J, editors. Critical Care Toxicology. Diagnosis and Management of the Critically Poisoned Patient. 2nd ed. Switzerland: Springer International Publishing AG; 2017. pp. 475-508

[48] Konca C, Yildizdas RD, Sari MY, Yükselmis U, Horoz OO, Yilmaz HL. Evaluation of children poisoned with calcium channel blocker or beta blocker drugs. Turkish Archives of Pediatrics. 2013;**48**:138-144. DOI: 10.4274/tpa.133

[49] Darracq MA, Thornton SL, Do HM, Bok D, Clark RF, Cantrell FL. Utilization of hyperinsulinemia euglycemia and intravenous fat emulsion following poison center recommendations. Journal of Medical Toxicology. 2013;**9**(3):226-230. DOI: 10.1007/s13181-013-0290-2

[50] Van Hare GF. Disturbances of rate and rhythm of the heart. In: Kliegman RM, Stanton BF, Schor NF, Geme JW St, Behram RE. Nelson Textbook of Pediatrics. 19th ed. Philadelphia, PA: Elsevier/Saunders; 2011. pp. 1610-1618

[51] Karturi SP, Gudmundsson H, Akhtar M, Jahangir A, Choudhuri I. Spectrum of cardiac manifestations from aconitine poisoning. HeartRhythm Case Reports. 2016;**2**(5):415-420. DOI: 10.1016/j.hrcr.2016.05.007

[52] Lee J, Czarnecki A, Hansen MS, Bucci C. Bidirectional ventricular tachycardia secondary to aconite toxicity after ingestion of a Chinese herbal supplement in Canada. International Journal of Case Reports and Images. 2018;**9**:1-4

[53] Tisdale JE. Drug-induced QT interval prolongation and torsades de pointes: Role of the pharmacist in risk assessment, prevention and management. Canadian Pharmacists Journal/Revue des Pharmaciens du Canada. 2016;**149**(3):139-151. DOI: 10.1177/1715163516641136

[54] Kawatou M, Masumoto H, Fukushima H, Morinaga G, Sakata R, Ashihara T, et al. Modelling torsade de pointes arrhythmias in vitro in 3D human iPS cell-engineered heart tissue. Nature Communications. 2017;**8**(1):1078. DOI: 10.1038/s41467-017-01125-y

[55] Kan AA, de Lange DW, Donker DW, Meulenbelt J. Management of prolonged QT interval and torsades de pointes in the intoxicated patient. The Netherlands Journal of Medicine. 2014;**72**(3):119-126

[56] Gosselin S, Jurlink DN, Kielstein JT, Ghannoum M, Lavergne V, Nolin TD, et al. Extracorporeal treatment for acetaminophen poisoning: Recommendations from the EXTRIP workgroup. Clinical Toxicology. 2014;**52**:856-867

[57] Ghannoun M, Hoffman RS, Gosellin S, Nolin TD, Lavergne V, Roberts DM. Use of extracorporeal treatments in the management of poisonings. Kidney International. 2018;**94**(4):682-688. DOI: 10.1016/j.kint.2018.03.026

[58] Saulnier F, Préau S, Onimus T, Six S, Durocher A. Épurations extracorporelles en toxicology Méd. Intensive Réa. 2016;**25**(5):514-528. DOI: DOI 10.1007/s13546-016-1218-z

[59] Mendonca S, Gupta S, Gupta A. Extracorporeal management of poisonings. Saudi Journal of Kidney Diseases and Transplantation. 2012;**23**(1):1-7

[60] Boyle M, Kurtovic J, Bihari D, Riordan S, Steiner C. Equipment review: The molecular adsorbents recirculating system (MARS®). Critical Care. 2004;**8**(4):280-286

[61] Covic A, Gusbeth-Tatomir VC, Goldsmith DJA. Molecular adsorbent recirculating system (MARS) dialysis for fulminant hepatic failure due to paracetamol overdose in children Mædica a. Journal of Clinical Medicine. 2006;**1**(2):11-15

[62] Pillukat MH, Schomacher T, Baier P, Gabriëls G, Pavenstädt H, HHJ S. Early initiation of MARS® dialysis in Amanita phalloides-induced acute liver injury prevents liver transplantation. Annals of Hepatology. 2016;**15**(5):775-787

[63] Lexmond WS, Van Dael CM, Scheenstra R, Goorhuis JF, Sieders E, Verkade HJ, et al. Experience with molecular adsorbent recirculating system treatment in 20 children listed for high-urgency liver transplantation. Liver Transplantation. 2015;**21**(3): 369-380. DOI: 10.1002/lt.24037

[64] Bergis D, Friedrich-Rust M, Zeuzem S, Betz C, Sarrazin C, Joerg Bojunga J. Treatment of amanita phalloides intoxication by fractionated plasma separation and adsorption (Prometheus®). Journal of Gastrointestinal and Liver Diseases. 2012;**21**(2):171-176

[65] Maiwall R, Maras JS, Nayak SL, Sarin SK. Liver dialysis in acute-on-chronic liver failure: Current and future perspectives. Hepatology International. 2014;**8**(Suppl 2):505-513. DOI: 10.1007/s12072-014-9534-8

[66] Hamdi T, Palmer BF. Review of extracorporeal membrane oxygenation and dialysis-based liver support devices for the use of nephrologists. American Journal of Nephrology. 2017;**46**:139-149. DOI: 10.1159/000479342

[67] Martínez JJG, Mollard F, Baud FJ, Bendjelid SK. Intoxication with calcium channel blockers and other highly protein bound drugs: Why use MARS? Two clinical case reports. Journal of Clinical Toxicology. 2018;**8**(3):1-7

[68] Mahongo CK, Grisoli D, Morera P, Jaussaud N, Lagier D, Collart F, et al. Intoxications médicamenteuses aiguës et ECMO, l'expérience marseillaise. Chirurgie Thoracique et Cardio-Vasculaire. 2015;**19**(4):228-233

[69] Wang GS, Levitan R, Wiegand TJ, Lowry J, Schult RF, Yin S. Extracorporeal membrane oxygenation (ECMO) for severe toxicological exposures: Review of the toxicology investigators consortium (ToxIC). Journal of Medical Toxicology. 2016;**12**:95-99

[70] Nakagawa TA, Stephen A, Mudit M, Stephen A, Mudit M, Mysore MR, et al. Guidelines for the determination of brain death in infants and children: An update of the 1987 task force recommendations. Pediatrics. 2011;**128**:e720-e740. DOI: 10.1542/peds.2011-1511

[71] Staple L, MacIntyre J, Murphy NG, Beed S. Organ and tissue donation from poisoned patients in the emergency department: A Canadian emergency physician survey. Canadian Journal of Emergency Medicine. 2018;**10**:1-8. DOI: 10.1017/cem.2018.43

[72] Karcioglu O. How to consider and manage brain death in a emergency

setting. Marmara Medical Journal. 2000;**13**(1):38-44

[73] Hanson P. Prélèvements d'organes chez un sujet décédé par intoxication. Quels risques? Urgences. 2010. Prelevements_d_organes_chez_un_sujet_decede_par_intoxication-_Quels_risques.pdf

[74] Natori Y. Legal determination of brain death. Japan Medical Association Journal. 2011;**54**(6):363-367

Chapter 3

# Forensic Toxicology

*Sahar Y. Issa*

## Abstract

Forensic toxicology is a broad science that integrates principles and practices about toxicology and legal aspects, which occur in conjunction with medicolegal instances as with homicide, suicide, road traffic and other types of accident and/or disasters. Nowadays, the practitioners of forensic toxicology science have to deal with three chief sections, namely: postmortem, drug testing, and human performance forensic toxicology. Postmortem forensic toxicology is dealing mostly with investigation of abnormal deaths, or when drug intoxication incidence is assumed as a cause of death and no abnormal findings were detected during autopsy.

**Keywords:** forensic toxicology, postmortem, workplace testing, drugs of abuse, adulteration

## 1. Introduction

Toxicology; is the study of the toxic effect of chemicals or xenobiotic on living organisms, particularly the humans, or animals. Toxicology involves studying the symptoms, mechanisms, detection and treatments of poisoning of a living body. Chemicals, or toxic agents, may be biological, physical, or chemical. As the toxicology and science are in a continuous evolving status, the familiarity to the effects of toxic agents on human body keeps progression and advancement [1].

Toxicology is usually referred to as the "science of poisons," including the continuous study of all toxic effects of physical or chemicals compounds and the association between the causative defined dose and its effect on any exposed body [2].

Habitually, the toxicology is defined as the science representing the information, source, toxic or fatal effect, lethal dose determination, analysis of poisons and the curative methods used to treat any of such exposures [1].

## 2. Some definitions

A poison is a chemical or substance that can induce damage or death when our bodies are exposed to, and it is only the optimum doses that can distinguish a poison from a therapeutic agent. All known chemicals can lead to cellular damage or death under certain circumstances and if they exceeded permissible or therapeutic ranges. Therefore, a poison can be defined as any substance capable of producing injurious effects in a living organism.

Toxicologists are the trained experts who can evaluate the role of toxic substances and their adverse effects on living organisms or environment [2, 3].

The broad spectrum of probable toxic adverse effects and the endless lists of chemicals existing in our environment, together make toxicology a very broad field of science. Consequently, many specialties of toxicology are needed to handle the numerous areas of toxicology science, including but not limited to; clinical, forensic, marine, and environmental toxicologists.

Forensics, by definition, is the use of science within the legal system to interpret a medical finding. The difference between clinical and forensic toxicology is not in the science or the methodologies used, but the difference lies in the end use of the attained results [4].

In clinical toxicology, the end user is a physician using the findings to treat and care for an intoxicated or poisoned patient, while in forensic toxicology, the end user can be a physician, a non-medical professional such as a lawyer, an employee, or police officer using the results to interpret a cause of death, employment eligibility, or compliance with workforce laws and terms. Hence, based on such situation the toxicologist may be a Physician, pharmacist, scientist, laboratory specialist or technician [3].

### 2.1 Main branches of toxicology

The professional activities of scientists and medical professionals within the field of toxicology fall into four main branches namely; forensic, industrial, clinical and environmental toxicology. Forensic toxicology is mainly concerned with the determination of the presence or absence and role of alcohol, drugs and their metabolites as well as other toxic substances in biological fluids, and/or tissues to solve a medico legal problem [5].

Based on that forensic toxicology is mainly referred to the science entailing the fusion of analytical forensic chemistry with toxicological principles and effects, dealing toxic substances, drugs of abuse, doping agents, chemical warfare agents, and their metabolisms and analyses, which are related to laws and ethics. Scientists responsible for testing bodily fluids and tissue samples during autopsies looking for the presence of chemicals, as well as laboratory specialists concerned with determination of presence or absence of any recreational drug or substance in samples collected from employees, or sportsmen are usually referred to as forensic toxicologists. Such toxicologists work mainly in laboratories to perform tests on samples collected by crime scene investigators, or workplace or sport officers [2–4].

Forensic toxicology laboratories handle the analytical procedures performed on both biological and sometimes non-biological samples to search for controlled substances. Following that, they generate analysis reports requested by the criminal justice system, or workforce departments. All Forensic Toxicology providers should exert sound efforts to guarantee that all their analytical results meet high ethical and moral standards and that all working personnel adhere to relevant legislation of the country [1].

The forensic toxicology laboratory should have standard operating procedures (SOPs) that are complete, updated, and accessible to all toxicologists carrying out forensic toxicology tests. SOPs should include detailed descriptions of all procedural processes starting from sample receiving, fulfillment of secured chain of custody, analysis, quality assurance and quality control (including validation of methods), reviewing of data, reporting and sample disposal as well as electronic program usage and security protocols of such programs if any. Their performance should be thoroughly and periodically assessed to accept the results released by their laboratories [3].

Forensic toxicology jobs most of the time involve testing for the presence of toxic gases (e.g., carbon monoxide, hydrogen sulfide, or phosphine); illegal or medicinal drugs; toxins; liquor; metals or elements; and other toxic substances when intoxication or drug poisoning are anticipated. Their scope of responsibility may include analyzing samples from criminal cases, and once their analytical reports are ready, they might present their testimony about it in a court of law [4].

Using highly specialized tests, methodologies and state-of-the-art equipment, chemical and biomedical instrumentation and chemical reagents, forensic toxicologists are requested to determine either the presence or the absence of chemicals while documenting each step of the process, and to determine the concentration of any detected substance to help finding out whether or not such xenobiotic was a cause of an unexplained death, accident or act [5].

The majority of forensic toxicologists are employed by law enforcement agencies, private drug testing facilities, and governmental bodies as Ministry of health in some countries. In forensic toxicology the main interest is the extent to which drugs and poisons may have contributed to impairment or death. In the field of forensic toxicology, the accreditation is important. It requires a great deal of energy and expense but does not, however, warranty all of the quality levels needed.

The conformity of a forensic toxicology laboratory with acknowledged quality and management structures is currently mandated in many countries, to be able to accept their analytical results and reports. As there are an essentially unlimited number of poisons that may be present in individual cases, therefore forensic toxicology is a scientific discipline in which everlasting efforts should be constantly exerted to complete and improve the methods of poison detection and show its close relation to raising quality [4–6].

Forensic toxicology can hence be generally divided into three main sectors [2–4]:

- *Workplace or pre-employment testing* dealing with pre-employment drug screens or drug screens required by the workplace.

- *Postmortem toxicology* dealing with the toxicology testing on deceased individuals and is a routine part of the autopsy process. Main aim is establishing the cause of death and clarifying its circumstances in postmortem investigation. Postmortem toxicology involves not only determining the presence and the amount of toxic substance in the postmortem body, but how the body's natural processes affect the substance, including chemical change and dilution.

- *Human performance testing* or Criminal Toxicology is used to elucidate the absence or presence of substances modifying human performance or behavior. This could be dealing with the determinants or toxicological factors in the investigation of criminal offenses, driving under the influence of alcohol or drugs, committing a crime while on a drug, or having a crime committed against an individual such as a sexual assault.

Therefore, the work of forensic toxicologist is considered as highly complicated as small quantities of poisons and their metabolites are to be isolated, purified and quantified from a highly complex matrix. Individual Forensic Toxicology specimens should be handled in such a manner as to reduce the possibility of degradation, contamination, adulteration, and/or damage during all steps from collection to transport, analysis and finally result reporting. Conventional transportation of specimens to the toxicology laboratory might include manual delivery, postal shipments, or a private courier service. A chain-of-custody form should be designed that will accompany specimens from the place of collection to the laboratory [7].

## 3. Workplace drug testing

Workplace drug testing is divided into two divisions, regulated and nonregulated testing:

- Regulated testing is testing that is mandated by the government via the Ministry of Health Services. This testing is mostly mandatory mainly for drivers, all governmental employees, military employees, and for those with many other jobs, in most of the countries.

- Non-regulated workplace drug testing is any testing that is required of a new employee to start a job, or it might be requested by workplace as random unplanned frequent screening for some workplaces as for pilots, workers in sensitive positions, or soldiers. The guidelines are not as strict as regulated testing, although the basic tenants are still adhered to [1].

### 3.1 Samples used for screening in workplace testing

#### *3.1.1 Urine sample*

The specimen for regulated workplace testing is always urine, but in some countries, an additional sample is requested, which might be oral fluid sample, or blood sample. It must be collected under direct observation or with measures in place so that tampering with the collection are eliminated, as by using adulteration detection kits directly after sample collection by donor, where the samples proved to be adulterated are rejected before being received by the laboratory personnel.

Secured chain of custody is applied for all samples collected since their collection till the release of the final Analytical report [7].

#### *3.1.2 Blood sample*

Blood sample is of particularly useful to the forensic toxicologists since the drug or poison existence in blood shows that exposure followed by absorption has taken place, hence a recent exposure might be ascertained. Furthermore, significant associations exist between the blood levels of most chemicals, poisons or drugs and their pharmacological and/or behavioral effects exerted on living bodies. On the other hand, urine drug levels, only indicate a previous drug exposure without conclusive evidence about the exact time of possible exposure or its probable physiological effects [4].

#### *3.1.3 Oral fluid sample*

Oral fluid is getting recent credit as a standard matrix for rapid drugs or substances of abuse detection. When compared to blood and urine samples, the oral fluid collection is non-invasive, easy technique with negligible intrusion into personal privacy. Such a sample can be collected under direct observation, consequently excluding the likelihood of sample exchange or adulteration as seen with urine samples. Hence, oral fluid can be beneficial in numerous situations that necessitate drug testing, as workplace screening, drug monitoring follow up, or for definitive treatment [2–4].

When compared to urine samples, oral fluid is a better reflection of blood concentrations of a drug. It specifies recent drug use and offers better association with pharmacological effects such as impaired driving performance. Hence, recently it is considered as the most appropriate biological matrix that enables roadside testing in road traffic accidents or other situations mandating the diagnosis of driving under the influence of drugs or alcohol.

It is becoming a more accepted testing specimen, due to the ease of its collection. Being an ideal specimen to collect where a restroom is not available, such as at the scene of a traffic accident, popularity of using oral fluid sample is increasing by time. As oral fluid is a hyper filtrate of blood, parent compounds are detected opposed to metabolites. Detection lengths are thus shorter than in urine, being only 1–2 days compared with 2–5 days with urine [7].

#### *3.1.4 Hair samples*

Hair is an alternative sample type that can be used for drug testing. The main advantage over the other samples is the wider length of detection, as in hair it might reach up to 3 months. However, environmental contamination is a major concern with hair testing, so laboratories must take special precautions during specimen preparations to ensure removal of environmental contamination.

#### *3.1.5 Human breath testing*

Lastly, another biological sample that has established recognition in many global areas in forensic toxicology testing is human breath. It is usually sampled for the detection and estimation of blood alcohol concentration in an individual and the detected level will be compared with the legal level of each country for driving under the effect of alcohol and other driving related offenses. It may also be sampled for the presence or absence of inhalants, most of which are volatile organic solvents that are not easily detected in blood, that are getting more abused among youths and adolescents [1–5].

### **3.2 Urine sample adulteration**

Specific precautions are required to determine if the specimen has been tampered with or adulterated in any way. All urine samples should be tested for creatinine, specific gravity, pH, and oxidants (nitrites).

When specimen adulteration testing falls out of the specified ranges of what is considered normal, it is termed as one of four classes, namely; diluted, substituted, adulterated, or invalid.

#### *3.2.1 Diluted sample*

A substituted specimen will be identified if [2–7]:

- The serum creatinine level exceeded 5 mg/dL or was below 20 mg/dL; and
- A specific gravity above 1.0010 or below 1.0030.

#### *3.2.2 Substituted sample*

Substituted sample is generally applied to non-human samples submitted by the donor during testing process. Any sample will be reported as substituted one if:

- The serum creatinine level was below 2 mg/dL; and
- The specific gravity is less than or equal to 1.0010 or greater than or equal to 1.0200.

### *3.2.3 Adulterated sample*

If the donor has added any substance to the collected sample, this will be referred to as an adulterated sample. Such sample should be reported as adulterated when any of the following criteria is encountered:

- pH < 3
- pH ≥ 11
- Nitrite ≥ 500 mg/mL
- Presence of chromium
- Presence of a bleach, iodine, or fluoride
- Presence of glutaraldehyde
- Presence of pyridine
- Detection of surfactant

### *3.2.4 Invalid sample*

A specimen will be reported as invalid when any of the following conditions is met:

- Creatinine concentration and specific gravity results are discrepant: Creatinine < 2 mg/dL and specific gravity > 1.0010 or < 1.0200
- Creatinine is ≥ 2 mg/dL and specific gravity is ≤ 1.0010.
- pH is outside the acceptable range: pH ≥ 3 and < 4.5
- pH ≥ 9 and < 11
- Nitrite ≥ 200 mg/mL and < 500 mg/mL.
- Urine that falls into any of these four categories is considered to have failed the drug test, even if the tests for drugs are all negative.

## 4. Postmortem testing

Analytical toxicology is a main procedure following the autopsy process. In postmortem setting and directly after death, metabolism of drugs and chemicals cease. If an autopsy is performed within a reasonable time frame, and the body was protected from harsh environmental conditions, the toxicology results will be as close as possible to what was in the body directly at the time of death. Quantitation of any drugs can indicate if an overdose occurred, a sub-therapeutic drug level was present, or a combination of multiple substances contributed to the cause of death [8].

In contrast to workplace drug testing, where urine samples are usually analyzed for a relatively fewer drugs and/or drug metabolites, the scope of work in postmortem forensic toxicology often encompasses search analysis for a larger number of poisons and drugs in numerous altered samples including blood, gastric contents, vitreous, and tissues including; renal, liver, spleen, muscle and brain tissues [5].

In addition, analysis of blood is mostly noteworthy as lethal drug concentrations in blood are well known for most of the drugs. However, drug concentrations in blood are generally lower than in urine or in tissues, which make their detection much harder than in urine samples [3, 5].

In many occasions, the forensic pathologist is dependent on the toxicological results to offer aid in determination of the cause of death. This is usually the situation when either gross or microscopic examinations during the autopsy process do not interpret a cause of death [9].

The forensic pathologists' requests of the forensic toxicologist have transformed over the last years. Before, they mainly requested identifying and reporting any lethal drug and/or poison levels that eventually lead to death. Definitely, due to the obvious limitations in the methods available at that time, this was the only possible request [10].

Accordingly, many drug-related deaths before were probably pass unobserved. But in modern times, larger scope of results and interpretations were requested from forensic toxicologists to clarify, including reporting drugs given at therapeutic or even sub therapeutic doses.

Such contribution might help to determine whether the deceased was compliant in taking the prescribed medicine. Many questions can be easily answered by toxicologists in current years as finding out whether noncompliance contributed to the death occurrence or not, or did the simultaneous use of many groups of medication together at therapeutic doses lead to unwanted drug interactions.

Another common question encountered by forensic pathologists is to clarify whether or not the deceased was under the effect of drugs at the time of the fatal accident, or was the suspect of the homicide under the influence of illegal drugs. Nowadays, such queries can best be easily answered by forensic toxicology laboratories equipped with state-of-the-art chromatographic instruments attached to mass spectroscopic units [1–3, 5].

### 4.1 Specimen

Postmortem testing is not limited to only urine. Specimens can be blood, urine, vitreous humor, gastric contents, liver tissue, hair, fingernails, or bile. This is not a comprehensive list. In postmortem investigations, the types of samples and tissue specimens and fluids needed for toxicological investigation are based often on the body condition and the type and/or number of analytes that must be identified and hence quantified. The toxicologist should also be informed about any putrefactive state of the body, injuries owing to the manner of death and other autopsy findings [3].

Many deaths involve ingestion of multiple drugs, necessitating larger amounts of tissue and fluids to be collected at post-mortem examination for toxicological examination. Prior to tissue extraction and analysis, all analyzed tissues must be homogenized. Water or buffer solutions such as sodium phosphate, might be added to the tissue sample preceding homogenization. It is vital to record the tissue weight as well as the fluid volume used to homogenize tissues in, as such data is of utmost importance in correctly estimate the drug concentration per each tissue weight unit [10].

Effective sample extraction and non-contamination are additional analytical process challenges while dealing with postmortem samples collected from decomposed bodies. Decomposition Products, can diminish the efficacy of extraction and produce interfering peaks during the analytical processes using chromatography methods. Also, tissue homogenates containing fatty materials must be separated from the drug analytes prior to analysis [1–3].

Basic drugs can be efficiently separated from lipid material by a process known as back-extraction, where the extracted drug from the tissue homogenate into a water-immiscible organic solvent and then back-extracted into a dilute acid solution where the neutral lipid material remains in the immiscible organic solvent, and the dilute acid solution will be turned basic to re-extracted the drug again into an organic solvent [1–3, 5].

All items collected from the death scene such as powders, pills, syringes, tools or liquids must be sent for analysis as well. A precise report including full description of the sample type and the site of collection should be prepared and sent to the laboratory with the samples needed to be analyzed. Blood samples can be collected from different body parts, as each area or collection compartment can have a varying drug concentration. Central blood samples can be collected from the heart, jugular, subclavian, and femoral veins, while blood collected from other sites is called peripheral compartment blood [2].

Preferably, blood samples must be collected from central and at least one peripheral site, to overcome the probability that any of these sites might be contaminated owing to different death manners. Blood is usually collected into preservative treated tubes, to stop further blood sample decomposition. Another important factor is that most of collected specimens are often stored for extended time periods. Samples' states might be deteriorated by bacteria, which might give erroneous results' interpretation mainly for ethanol levels. Based on putrefactive state and manner of death, certain specimens may become contaminated with bacteria, either via exposure to the normal flora or through external contamination, as in case of a body with multiple open wounds or gunshots. The collection of specimens as well as the testing of these samples should always be performed under chain of custody. Postmortem blood is difficult to work with as a result of coagulation and/or degradation, and because of the state of the specimen at the time of testing [11].

### 4.2 Specimen type, amount and site of collection

The following is a suggested list of specimens and amounts to be collected at post-mortem in such cases [3–6, 9]:

- Femoral blood: at least 10 mL (site specified and suitably isolated).
- Urine: all available sample.
- Vitreous humor: all collected sample.
- Cavity/heart blood: not less than 25 mL, collected only if femoral blood is limited or not available.
- Hair: to be collected at the start of the autopsy prior to body evisceration.
- Bile sample: 10 mL.
- Liver, renal and/or spleen tissues: 10–20 g, mainly if low volume of blood available.
- Stomach contents: all available and any examples of undigested tablets/drug material (including potential plant toxin material.
- Brain tissue: 10–20 g (for volatiles).
- Lung tissue: 10–20 g (for volatiles).

- Samples collected by in health care facilities prior to death (ante mortem specimens) are samples of greater importance.

- Non-human items collected at the from death scene, which may have contributed to the death are considered as samples of utmost importance, in toxicological investigation in postmortem cases.

## 5. Human performance testing

How an individual acts when under the effect of a substance or drug of abuse is determined by human performance testing. This type of testing includes determination of blood alcohol level and drugs of abuse testing from a suspected driver. Blood testing for drugs from a potential drug assisted sexual assault, or testing of a worker exhibiting weird behavior while at work is another aspect of human performance testing. Criminal Toxicology is another aspect of human performance testing, where the determining factors or toxicological causes during the investigation of any criminal offenses have to be studied [12].

### 5.1 Specimen

The specimen of choice in human performance testing is blood, though oral fluid sample is another promising sample. Analyzing a blood sample is of utmost importance because upon confirming the presence of any abused substance, it is then probable to establish an estimated time frame of drug or substance exposure. Such finding is not likely to be estimated upon using a urine sample, where all drugs have a much longer detection window. Ability to conclusively verify the timeframe of drug consumption, is crucial in all human performance testing settings [3].

## 6. Types of testing in the field of forensic toxicology

### 6.1 Screening or initial testing

Initial testing of collected specimens, is known as screening or screen testing. It is done by immunoassay methods. The cutoffs to determine negative from nonnegative samples are established by Governmental regulatory bodies in each country. Any value greater than or equal to the cutoff is considered "nonnegative" (The term positive can only be used with confirmatory testing because of the possibility of false-positive screening test). Screening testing is done for a specific class of drugs; opiates, amphetamines, benzodiazepines, etc.

If all performed initial screening tests were negative, the results will be released as negative and there is no further testing to be requested. If any of the performed test results were equal to or above the cutoff value, a new aliquot from the main sample will be obtained and confirmatory testing will be started.

The initial identification or detection of drugs and other toxins by an immunoassay or enzymatic screening methods should be confirmed by a second procedure utilizing a different analytical principle. It is to be well stated that the use of a second immunoassay screening system (e.g. RIA—radioimmunoassay) to confirm another immunoassay result (e.g. FPIA—fluorescence polarization immunoassay), is not acceptable, even if it is supposed to be a more specific assay or testing procedure. Final results are not released until all confirmatory results are finalized [13].

### 6.2 Confirmatory testing

The forensic toxicologist is usually confronted with the hard mission of screening a given sample for the “unknown”. The toxicology laboratory consequently must be equipped with state-of-the-art instruments, capable enough to perform a wide range of toxicological tests with high specificity. This procedure is usually referred to as “systematic toxicological analysis” (STA), or “general unknown screening”.

All chemical substances exposed to screening procedures, must be firstly separated from the liquidified biological matrix. The simplest sample preparation method is to use a water miscible solvent, as acetonitrile or acetone. Such solvents will be added to the biological fluid to precipitate protein and other unwanted constituents. A filtration or centrifugation step follows before the extraction processes that end up with a more concentrated extract than the original sample, followed by the final confirmatory analytical step.

Confirmation testing is performed by detector as mass spectrometry, coupled either to Chromatography technique that provides a chemical separation of analytes in a gaseous (GC) or liquid (LC) system namely; gas chromatography or liquid chromatography. The selected detector should be appropriate to the analytes among other factors. The testing occurs on a fresh aliquot from the original sample, to exclude likelihood of a possible erroneously mix up with the initial screening aliquot [11].

For each drug class to be screened, there is a group of specific confirmatory tests. Such analytical confirmatory testing result is conclusive, and indisputable, when the testing process is performed correctly. Such an assurance is partly based on the fact that the confirmed result was reached based on multiple parameters, e.g.; retention times, parent and daughter ions ratios. If confirmatory testing procedure is performed correctly and properly maintained through applying proficiency testing with similar laboratories, the confirmation test is considered to be definitive and undisputable [9].

## 7. Result reporting

Reporting of the results is done following a second review of all results by another laboratory personnel who was not a part of the testing process. On finding them acceptable, all results will be certified and released either to the medical review officer or to the requesting entity [1–3].

A medical review officer is usually a physician acting as an intermediary between the Toxicology laboratory and the requestor or client who ordered for the test. The medical review officer should be well trained to communicate with the client, donor, and legal representative and/or forensic pathologist to help interpreting the testing results. They are responsible to deal with a donor whose samples proved to be positive, and determine if the detected drug was taken complying with a physician’s instructions or were recreationally abused [5–7].

Following the release of a final report, it might turn out to be essential to correct an error that might be typographical or otherwise. A corrected report should be issued in this occasion comprising the same demographic data as in the original report(s) and be well labeled as a corrected report replacing the original faulty one.

Forwarding samples to another laboratory for analysis or result evaluation, should be well recorded and referred to on the final report/statement demonstrating this fact. Results of referred laboratory tests may be integrated into the original laboratory’s final report/statement, but the name of the laboratory that truly carried out the test should be clearly stated [1–4].

## 8. Accreditation

Forensic toxicology laboratory accreditation is an important recommendation to standardize the results. Proficiency testing and comparing results to certified regional laboratories is an initial step during the journey to laboratory accreditation [3, 5–8].

## Conflict of interest

No conflict or competing of interests to declare.

## Thanks

"I have to start by thanking my awesome husband, Mohammed. From reading early drafts of my chapter to giving me advice on the scientific content to taking care of Yasmin and Yousef our young daughter and son so I could edit, he was as important to this book chapter getting done as I was. Thank you so much, dear."

"Thanks to everyone on the IntechOpen team who helped me so much. Special thanks to Martina Josavac, the ever-patient Author Service Manager for her great help."

## Acronyms and abbreviations

| | |
|---|---|
| GC | gas chromatography |
| FPIA | fluorescence polarization immunoassay |
| LC | liquid chromatography |
| RIA | radioimmunoassay |
| SOPs | standard operating procedures |
| STA | systematic toxicological analysis |

## Author details

Sahar Y. Issa
Faculty of Medicine, Alexandria University, Egypt

*Address all correspondence to: sahar_issa71@yahoo.com

## References

[1] Smith MP, Bluth MH. Forensic toxicology. Clinics in Laboratory Medicine. Dec 2016;**36**(4):753-759

[2] Chris Kostakis, Peter Harpas, Peter C. Stockham, Chapter 11 - Forensic toxicology, Editor(s): Salvatore Fanali, Paul R. Haddad, Colin F. Poole, Marja-Liisa Riekkola. In: Liquid Chromatography (Second Edition). Elsevier; 2017. Pages 301-358

[3] Cosbey S, Elliott S, Paterson S. The United Kingdom and Ireland Association of Forensic Toxicologists; establishing best practice for professional training & development in forensic toxicology. Science & Justice: Journal of the Forensic Science Society. 2017;**57**(1):63-71

[4] Drug Enforcement Administration, Department of Justice. Schedules of controlled substances: Extension of temporary placement of UR-144, XLR11, and AKB48 in schedule I of the Controlled Substances Act. Final order. Federal Register. 2015;**80**(94):27854-27856

[5] Jones JT. Advances in drug testing for substance abuse alternative programs. Journal of Nursing Regulation. 2016;**6**(4):62-67

[6] Elliott SP, Stephen DWS, Paterson S. The United Kingdom and Ireland association of forensic toxicologists forensic toxicology laboratory guidelines. Science & Justice. Sep 2018;**58**(5):335-345

[7] US Department of Health and Human Services, Substance Abuse and Mental Health Services Administration. Medical Review Officer Manual for Federal Agency Workplace Drug Testing Programs. Rockville (MD): Substance Abuse and Mental Health Services Administration; 2010

[8] Levine B. Postmortem forensic toxicology. In: Levine B, editor. Principles of Forensic Toxicology. 3rd ed. Washington, DC: AACC Press; 2009. pp. 3-13

[9] Committee on Identifying the Needs of the Forensic Sciences Community, National Research Council. Strengthening Forensic Science in the United States: A Path Forward. Washington (DC): National Academies Press; 2009

[10] Kunsman GW. Human performance toxicology. In: Levine B, editor. Principles of Forensic Toxicology. 3rd ed. Washington, DC: AACC Press; 2009. pp. 15-29

[11] Hedlund J, Forsman J, Sturup J, Masterman T. Pre-offense alcohol intake in homicide offenders and victims: A forensic toxicological case-control study. Journal of Forensic and Legal Medicine. 2018;**56**:55-58

[12] Dinis-Oliveira RJ, Carvalho F, Duarte JA, et al. Collection of biological samples in forensic toxicology. Toxicology Mechanisms and Methods. 2010;**20**(7):363-414

Section 2

# Organ-Specific Effects and Toxicological Agents

Chapter 4

# Review of Health Hazards and Toxicological Effects of Constituents of Cosmetics

*John Kanayochukwu Nduka, Henrietta Ijeoma Kelle and Isaac Omoche Odiba*

## Abstract

Cosmetic products are designed for use on human body for beautifying and promoting attractiveness and appearance; for these reasons, cosmetics are in high demand especially among women of all ages in every country. Despite many vulnerabilities associated with cosmetic usage, the cosmetic and 'makeup' continues to enjoy wide acceptability irrespective of age and sex. This is made possible by massive advertising employed by producers and marketers of cosmetics. Advertising is the link between manufactured products and would-be consumers; it plays a crucial role in determining the product that is mostly patronised and vice versa. Therefore, ethical advertising that promotes utilitarian benefits of cosmetics should be encouraged over and above emotional advertisement that lowers self-esteem of consumers and offers such products as solution to their low self-esteem. Despite the ban in many countries of poisonous substances in cosmetic products, inexhaustive list of substances, such as lead, chromium, nickel, mercury, arsenic, cadmium, hydroquinone, steroids, nitrosamine, etc. are still present in many cosmetic products. In most cases, above regulatory values, cancers, renal disorders, thinning and easy brushing of the skin, dermatophyte infection with lesions, macular hyper pigmentation, pityriasis vesicular, diabetes mellitus, micropapular eruption, hypertension, etc. are possible toxicological and health hazards that may be associated with continuous cosmetic application.

**Keywords:** cosmetics, hazardous constituents, toxicological effects, public health issues, continuous cosmetic usage

## 1. Introduction

Body and personal care products (cosmetics) are designed to be applied on body parts for the purpose of enhancing cleaning, protecting, beautifying, healthy and young looking appearance or altering appearance without changing the body's operational nature [1, 2]. Body care products are of different kinds like skin moisturizers, perfumes, lipsticks and lip glosses, finger nail polishes, eye and facial makeup preparations, shampoo, hair colours and deodorant [3, 4]. A distinction that is made between cosmetics and drugs is that the latter is described as substances used as medicine or used in medicine. That is, drugs are intended to be used to treat or prevent ailments or diseases upon reaction with the human system. In addition, unlike cosmetics, drugs must be subjected to and pass premarket screening test(s) where they are proven to be safe and effective before they are marketed [3]. Certain chemicals that are part of cosmetic formulations have been found to be harmful, and the usage of cosmetic products containing such chemicals portends danger for human health. Inexhaustive list include heavy metals, hydroquinone, steroids, phenols and nitrosamines, etc. [1, 2, 5–9]. Surprisingly, in spite of the regulations put in place to prevent or minimize the presence of such ingredients in cosmetic brands, heavy metals, organic and inorganic chemical substances are still very much in them. A reason given for this is that such substances may be a major component of the raw materials used in cosmetic manufacture or are deliberately included in cosmetics [1, 6].

Cosmetic products appear not to be subjected to clinical trials or laboratory testing(s) by regulatory authority in Nigeria before premarket approval. This is evident from legal document setting up the Nigerian National Agency for Food and Drug Administration and Control (NAFDAC). Guidelines stating the necessary requirement for registration of imported cosmetics in Nigeria are the attachment of certificate of analysis to the application for registration. This implies that safety and quality of products are monitored through post-market surveillance (PMS) activity. The implication is that laboratory/clinical testing of cosmetic products by NAFDAC takes place only when a victim of hazardous effect of cosmetic is reported or an end user discovers it to be defective or have side effects on the consumers. The guidelines prohibit mercury and its compounds, including corticosteroids. The reason is that mercury is a known cause of dermatitis and kidney damage which could manifest as hypertension. Continuous and possible excessive application of corticosteroids through cosmetics on the skin is reported to cause recalcitrant acne, red striae, excessive hairiness, proneness to infections, insulin related ailments and cataract [10]. Creams with hydroquinone at a concentration higher or in amount in excess of two percent (2%) are under prohibition because their side effect manifests as exogenous ochronosis which is depicted as a dirty brown pigmentation or colouration on areas of the body exposed to the sun followed by the skin's loss of elasticity [10].

The cosmetic market in Nigeria is currently flooded with a variety of cosmetic products in response to the high demands for such products [7]. Nigeria with a conservative population estimated at 154,774,091 people as in February 2010 [11] whose citizens are regarded as being highly fashionable and glamorous provides an ever increasing market for cosmetic product manufacture, marketers and importers. Cosmetic manufacturers and marketers/distributors selling products containing mercury and corticosteroids usually violate fair packaging and labelling requirements by not always listing them as ingredients of the products. Furthermore, dark-skinned African populace use cosmetic majorly in an attempt to change their skin colour in response to social pressures [7]. Society tends to associate affluence (social and professional success) with physical attractiveness [12]. This may suggest the rationale behind the advertising strategy of most cosmetic manufacturers and marketers whereby their products are promoted majorly by exposing the populace to pictures of good-looking and even slightly above-average-looking females [3, 12]. It may also suggest the reason why Nigerian women were ranked high on a list of African countries known for patronizing skin lightening products [6].

Nigeria, irrespective of their social-economic background, attach a lot of importance to their looks and actively seek to improve such regardless of the cost or implications [7].

Although skin lightening products alter the body's structure and function by inhibiting and/or reducing melanogenesis [2, 6, 9, 13], they are classified as cosmetics rather than drugs and can be readily purchased over the counter at roadside non-pharmaceutical stores. As a result, these products are much more readily available, and since some of them come very cheap, anybody, regardless of socio-economic background would always find a product that is affordable [7]. The choice of product usage is compounded by ignorance, illiteracy and make-believe lifestyle. According to the Nigeria's National Literacy Survey [11] carried out by Nigeria's National Bureau of Statistics, the study revealed that the adult literacy level rate in English language stands at 57.9%. This makes it difficult for a large segment of the population (42.1%) to even read and comprehend the inscriptions on the label of cosmetic product, leaving them ignorant of the actual benefits and risks associated with the cosmetics they have decided to use. That aside, the quest for survival makes even the literate populace to pay little attention to information on content and instruction on direction of use that are contained on the product labels. A huge chunk of the cosmetic brands found in Nigeria are imported from America, Europe and Asia. It is not surprising, as Nigerians view products tagged 'foreign' as being of superior quality and therefore attach greater value to such products than locally manufactured ones. In order to maintain a clean and healthy environment that is free of pollution as well as protects public health, potential public health and environmental pollutant such as cosmetics must have their contents carefully and properly scrutinized and continuously monitored. The aim of this review is to X-ray the toxicological profile and effects of toxicants contained in cosmetic brands in Nigerian market and elsewhere.

## 2. Types of cosmetics

Many cosmetic products exist in Nigerian market and elsewhere across the globe; some are locally made, while others are imported. They may occur in liquid, semi-liquid, solid, granular and volatile form; examples include skincare creams, hair creams, toothpaste, soaps, perfumes, lipsticks, fingernail and the toe polish, eye and facial makeup, towelettes, permanent waves, hair colours, hair sprays and gels, deodorants, hand sanitizer, etc. [3]. A 'make-up is a micro aspect of cosmetics', which ordinarily can refer to colouring products intended to improve the user's appearance.

## 3. Harmful substances in cosmetics

The presence of some substances in cosmetics constitutes imminent danger to the users. Such substances that may cause damage to the users of cosmetics include but not only:

### 3.1 Inorganic-heavy metals

These are metals having a specific gravity greater than four (4). Sulphides of such metals are insoluble in water. Examples of heavy metals are cadmium, lead, nickel, mercury, manganese, chromium, thallium, etc. [14].

### 3.2 Arsenic (As)

Arsenic occurs in many minerals, in conjunction with sulphur and other metals, and also as a pure elemental crystal. Arsenic is a metalloid. It can exist in various allotropes, although only the grey form has important use in industry [15]. It is notoriously poisonous to multicellular life, although a few species of bacteria are able to use arsenic compounds as respiratory metabolites. Arsenic contamination of groundwater is a problem that affects millions of people across the globe [16].

### 3.3 Cadmium (Cd)

Cadmium belongs to group IIB (group 12) of the periodic table and is used in nickel-cadmium storage battery where it enhances long service life and a wide operating range. It occurs in nature mostly in zinc deposits in the mineral greenockite (CdS) and otavite ($CdCO_3$). Its abundance in the earth's crust is estimated to be 0.15 mg/kg and in sea water 0.11 μg/L [17].

### 3.4 Lead (Pb)

Lead belongs to group IVA (group 14) of the periodic table. It is one of the oldest metals known to civilization. It is rarely found in nature in its native form but can be found in several minerals such as galena (PbS), angelsite ($PbSO_4$) and cerussite ($PbCO_3$). Its concentration in the earth's crust is 12.5 mg/kg and in sea water, 0.03 mg/L [17]. Lead and its alloys such as solder can be used in the construction of pipelines, plumbing fixtures, wires, ammunition, containers for corrosive acids and shield against short wavelength radiation.

### 3.5 Nickel (Ni)

Nickel is a transition metal, the most common oxidation state is +2, abundance in the earth crust is 84 μg/kg, and its average concentration in seawater is 0.56 μg/mL. It occurs in nature as in pentlandite $(NiFe)_9S_{16}$, limonite $(FeNi)O(OH).nH_2O$ and garnierite $(NiMg)_6Si_4O_{10}(OH)_8$ [17]. Nickel metal is used in numerous alloys that are used to construct various equipment such as reaction vessels, plumbing parts, missiles and aerospace components. It is also used in catalysis [15].

### 3.6 Chromium (Cr)

Chromium belongs to group VIB (group 6) in the periodic table as a transition metal [15]. Chromium occurs in the mineral chromite, ($FeO.Cr_2O_3$), and its abundance in the earth's crust is estimated to be near 0.01%, and its concentration in sea water is 0.3 μg/L [17]. Its most important application is in the production of nickel-based alloys. Trace amounts of Cr are necessary in the diet of mammals. $Cr^{3+}$ and insulin are both involved in maintaining the correct level of glucose in the blood. In cases of Cr deficiency, glucose is only removed from the blood half as fast as normal. Some cases of diabetes may reflect faulty metabolism of Cr [15].

### 3.7 Manganese (Mn)

Manganese is distributed widely in nature, mostly as oxide, silicate and carbonate ores. It is the 12th most abundant element in the earth's crust. Its earth crust concentration is estimated to be 0.093%; average concentration in sea water is 2 μg/L. Most important industrial use is in ferrous metallurgy yet an essential element for plants and animals [17].

### 3.8 Mercury (Hg)

Mercury is the only liquid metal at standard temperature and pressure (STP), with a freezing point of −38.83°C and boiling point of 356.73°C; mercury has one of the narrowest ranges of its liquid state of any metal [18–20]. Mercury poisoning results from exposure to water-soluble forms of mercury (such as mercuric chloride or methylmercury), inhalation of mercury vapour, or eating seafood contaminated with mercury [15].

It is used in the manufacture of industrial chemicals, in electrical and electronic applications and in thermometers, especially when high temperatures are required. Larger proportions of gaseous mercury are used in fluorescent lamps, but its other applications are gradually replaced considering health and safety implications and in some applications totally substituted with less toxic but highly expensive Galinstan alloy [21].

Compounds of mercury have found extensive application in medicine but are much less utilized nowadays than previously intended, since its toxic effects are more widely understood. The element mercury is an ingredient in dental amalgams. Thiomersal (called Thimerosal in the United States) is an organic compound used as a preservative in vaccines, though it has declined remarkably [22]. Another mercury compound merbromin (mercurochrome) is a topical antiseptic used for minor cuts and scrapes and is still in use in some countries. In the 1930s, some vaccines were preserved with thiomersal, which can convert to ethyl mercury on degradation or metabolism. Although it was generally speculated that this mercury-based compound (preservative) can cause autism in children, scientific proof to support the speculation was lacking (Parker et al., 2004). But as a precautionary measure, the US government has removed or drastically reduced thiomersal in all US vaccines recommended for children 6 years of age or below, with the exception of inactivated influenza vaccine [22].

Cinnabar, a mercury compound, was utilized in traditional Chinese medicines. When its safety considerations were reviewed, it was found that it can cause serious mercury intoxication on application of heat, taken in more required concentration or on continuous exposure time, and can have adverse effects at therapeutic doses, though this is typically reversible at therapeutic doses. Despite the fact that mercury in this form may be less toxic than others, its utilization in traditional Chinese medicine can be justified as the therapeutic basis for the use has not been proved [23]. Presently, its application in medicine has slowed greatly in all aspect, especially in developed countries. Some over-the-counter drugs such as topical antiseptics, stimulants, laxatives, diaper-rash ointment and eye drops contain mercury compounds. The FDA has inadequate data to establish general recognition of the safety and effectiveness of the mercury ingredients in these products [22].

Thiomersal is widely used in the manufacture of mascara. In 2008, Minnesota in the United States became the first state to ban intentional use of mercury in cosmetics [24]. A study of mean concentration of mercury in urine samples shows skincare products as a major exposure route to inorganic mercury among New York City residents. Population-based bio-monitoring confirms sea food and fish meals as a major source of mercury [25]. Mercury can be absorbed through the skin and mucous membranes, while the vapours can be inhaled, so containers of mercury are securely sealed to avoid spills and evaporation. Literature has shown that the most toxic forms of mercury are its organic compounds, such as dimethylmercury and methylmercury. Inorganic compounds are highly toxic by ingestion or inhalation [26].

### 3.9 Nitrosamines

Nitrosamines are compounds of the chemical structure $R_1N\ (—R_2)—N=O$, most of which are carcinogenic. They are formed when secondary amines react with nitrous acid (generated by action of dilute acid on nitrites) in an environment with pH values below 7 [27]. They are used in the manufacture of some cosmetics, in pesticides and in most rubber products. In 1956, two British scientists, John Barnes and Peter Magee, reported that dimethylnitrosamine produced liver tumours in rats. Research was undertaken, and approximately 90% of nitrosamine compounds were deemed to be carcinogenic [28]. In the 1970s, increased frequency of liver cancer was found in Norwegian farm animals that were fed on herring meal that was preserved using sodium nitrite. The sodium nitrite had interacted with dimethylamine in the fish and produced dimethylnitrosamine [28].

### 3.10 Nitrite

Nitrite is the univalent radical $NO_2^-$ with a molecular weight of 46 g/mol or a compound containing it, such as a salt or an ester of nitrous acid [29]. The nitrite ion $NO_2^-$ has a V-shape that is based on a plane triangular structure; with nitrogen [N] at the centre, two corners are occupied by oxygen [O] atoms, and the third corner occupied by a lone pair. As a result, the N atom is $sp^2$ hybridized [15]. Nitrite is a weak oxidizing agent that oxidizes $Fe^{2+}$ to $Fe^{3+}$ and $I^-$ to $I_2$, while it is reduced to $N_2O$ or NO.

## 4. Organic substances

### 4.1 Hydroquinone

Hydroquinone, known as benzene-1,4-diol or quinol, is an aromatic organic compound that is a type of phenol. Its chemical structure features two hydroxyl groups bonded to a benzene ring in a para position. In a substituted form, the derivatives of the compound can still be referred to as hydroquinone.

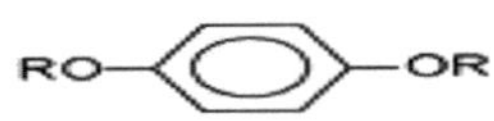


Hydroquinone (R = H)
Hydroquinone bis(trimethylsilyl ether) (R = $Si(CH_3)_3$)

Since it is weakly acidic, the reactivity of O—H groups of these compounds compares well with other phenols. Its conjugate base can easily undergo O-alkylation as to produce mono- and diethers. In the same way, hydroquinone is highly susceptible to ring substitution by Friedel-Crafts reactions such as alkylation. This reaction is used to produce much known antioxidants such as 2-tert-butyl-4-methoxyphenol ('BHA'). A very important dye quinizarin is produced by diacylation reaction of hydroquinone with phthalic anhydride [30], but the most important reaction is the conversion of hydroquinone to produce mono- and diamino derivatives—methylaminophenol, used in photography.

$$C_6H_4\,(OH)_2 + CH_3NH_2 \rightarrow C_6H_4\,(OH)\,(N\,(H)\,CH3) + H_2O \qquad (1)$$

Also diamines, useful in the rubber industry as antiozone agents, can be produced from aniline:

$$C_6H_4\,(OH)_2 + 2C_6H_5NH_2 \rightarrow C_6H_4\,(N\,(H)\,C_6H_5)_2 + 2\,H_2O \qquad (2)$$

The compound is variously used, mainly with its action as a reducing agent that dissolves in water. It is widely used in most photographic development for film and paper. It can act as an inhibitor by preventing polymerization of acrylic acid, methyl methacrylate, cyanoacrylate and other monomers that can respond to free radical-initiated joining. This reaction utilizes the antioxidant properties of hydroquinone to undergo mild oxidation and convert to the compound parabenzoquinone, $C_6H_4O_2$, often called p-quinone or quinone. This reaction is reversible as reduction of quinone reverses this reaction back to the original form. Some biochemical compounds in nature have this sort of hydroquinone or quinone section in their structures, such as coenzyme Q, and can undergo similar redox interconversions. Hydroquinone can lose an $H^+$ from both hydroxyl groups to form a diphenolate ion.

### 4.2 Steroids

This is an organic compound in which four cycloalkane rings are joined with each other; dietary fat cholesterol, the sex hormone—estradiol, testosterone and the anti-inflammatory drug dexamethasone are common examples. The steroid centre consists of 20 carbon atoms which are bound together where they exhibit the structure of 4 fused rings composed of 3 cyclohexane rings and 1 cyclopentane ring. They vary by the functional groups attached to this four-ring core and by the oxidation state of the rings [31]. All steroids are made in cells either from the sterol lanosterol (animals and fungi) or from cycloartenol (plants). Both lanosterol and cycloartenol are derived from the cyclization of the triterpene squalene [32].

Corticosteroids are a class of chemicals that includes steroid hormones naturally produced in the adrenal cortex of vertebrates and are involved in a wide range of physiological processes, including stress and immune response, and regulation of inflammation, carbohydrate metabolism and catabolism of protein. Synthetic glucocorticoids are used in the treatment of joint pain or inflammation, temporal arthritis, dermatitis, allergic reactions, asthma, hepatitis, systemic lupus erythematosus, ulcerative colitis, Crohn's disease and sarcoidosis and for glucocorticoid replacement or other forms of adrenal insufficiency (Higashi et al., 2009).

## 5. Bibliographies that prove cosmetic brands are in continuous use and contain poisonous toxicants

An epidemiological survey was conducted by Adebajo [7] on the use of skin lightening cosmetics among traders in Lagos, Nigeria, using 450 traders from three major and popular markets (Tejuosho, Balogun and Mushin) in Lagos metropolis between May and July 1998 using stratified sampling method. Information on their socio-demographic characteristics, knowledge and attitudes to and the patterns of use of skin lightening cosmetics were elicited from the respondents with the application of questionnaire-based interview. The result obtained showed that for socio-demographic characteristics of the respondents that participated, 28.9% were males and 71.1% females. 51.6% were aged between 20 and 29 years with a mean of 30.8 years and about 49.3% were married. Over 95% of the respondents had some form of formal education with 31.1% who had at least primary school education and 119 post-secondary school education. Most of them (82.2%) were traders, while the remaining operated small-scale business such as hairdressing, barbing, tailoring and chemist. Many of them (45.6%) earned less than N1, 000.00, while 18 (4.0%) earned above N5, 000.00 per month. For patterns of use of skin lightening cosmetics, 348 respondents (77.3%) made up of 96 male traders (27.6%) and 252 female traders (72.4%) admitted using skin lightening cosmetics. Sex did not have any effect on the pattern of use of these cosmetics ($p > 0.05$). Hydroquinone-based cosmetics were the most widely used by the respondents, and the least use was the mercury-based ones; female traders generally tended to use more corticosteroid-based cosmetics much more than male traders. The modal duration of the use of the skin lightening cosmetics was 1–3 years, although 29 respondents (8.3%) had used them for less than 6 months and 44 (12.6%) for 5 years. Many of the respondents (45.7%) who admitted using the cosmetics spent between N250 and N500 per month on the cosmetics, while some

(12.4%) spent between N500 and N1000. Over half of the respondent claimed that they discovered the skin lightening cosmetics themselves, while, 123 (35.3%) were influenced by their friends. Other sources of influence include health workers (2.3%), chemist (5.5%), parents (1.4%) and the media (1.4%). One hundred and nine respondents (31.3%) commenced the use of skin lightening cosmetics to treat skin blemishes. Almost one-third of the respondents (30.2%) indulged in the use of these cosmetics because they felt that being fair complexioned made them more attractive. Others use them to cleanse or tone their faces and bodies (21.0%), and the rest used them simply because they felt it was trendy to be fair complexioned. Only 14 respondents indulged in the use of skin lightening cosmetics to satisfy the desires of the opposite sex. Although the level of the use of skin lightening cosmetics increased with the level of education of the respondent, this was weakly significant ($p = 0.05$). One hundred and sixty seven (73.2%) Christians compared with 181 (81.5%) Moslems used bleaching creams. This difference was statistically significant ($p < 0.05$). On how respondents felt about their new look, most of the respondents (64.1%) felt they were more attractive; hence, they were more confident about their new look. Only 46 (13.2%) claimed they were relieved of their skin blemishes, while 33 (9.5%) were better appreciated by their spouses. About 50% of 348 respondents (made up of 44 males and 130 females) who use skin lightening cosmetics developed side effects. Respondents were more likely to develop side effects as duration of use increased from 6 months to 3 years. Beyond 3 years, however, fewer respondents developed side effects. The respondents reported several side effects, the commonest being yellowish brown colouration of the skin (23.9%). Others were skin rashes, multiple stretch marks, thinning and easy brushing of the skin. Twenty-five of the participants had worsening of their existing skin conditions, and on observing some of the side effects, 79 respondents (45.4%) just simply ignored the side effects, while only 35.6% stopped using the cosmetics. To mitigate against these problems, clinical trials should be conducted to ascertain the safety levels acceptable for the Nigerian skin types and climate.

Nnorom et al. [8] analysed the content of trace metal of several cosmetics in Nigeria for the presence of lead, cadmium, zinc and iron; three groups of facial cosmetics were used, such as eye pencil, eye liners and mascara, lipstick and lip gloss and native eyeliner (tiro and uhie) which were purchased from retail outlet and open market in Umuahia, Southeast Nigeria. The result from this study showed that the range of Pb levels for lipsticks is higher in concentration than that for local eyeliners, with the geometric mean value for the local eyeliners being 120.5 μg/g. Comparative amounts of Pb were found in the local eyeliners and pencil. Cd was generally low, being much less than 3 μg/g, while chromium was much higher than the corresponding levels of nickel and cadmium in each sample group. Cr, Fe and Zn were much higher in the samples than those of the non-essential metals, Pb, Ni and Cd. Zinc and Fe were in the highest concentration. The research concluded that the continuous use of these cosmetics could result in an increase in the trace metal levels in human body beyond acceptable limits.

Nnoruka and Okoye [9] studied topical steroid abuse to document the prevalence, motives and observed complications of steroid use as depigmenting agent among African Blacks of Southeast Nigeria; consecutively new patients are attending the dermatological clinic of the University of Nigeria Teaching Hospital, Enugu. Nigeria, from June to December 2004, was recruited. All the participants were adults (males and females) and were recruited only if they use depigmenting agents. These was ascertained by obtaining information from the back of the containers or packets of waste containers; leaflets containing useful information concerning active ingredients were used to ascertain that the products contained well-known active lightening substances such as hydroquinone, mercury compounds and steroids. Questionnaire was used to obtain information on the most frequently used cosmetic and mode of application with full consent of the patients. Relevant information such as age, sex, occupation, demographic information as well as names and types of products utilized within the last three months; length of and regularity of application and body parts involved; amount or volume utilized monthly and cost involved were determined. Also medical history of the patients, if they have had other medical conditions such as hypertension, diabetes mellitus or renal disorders, and the duration of such problems. Manner and method of presenting the problem and clinical examination already are carried out in the affected areas. Where adequate information were not obtained or unsatisfactory, relevant laboratory tests like mycological studies, venereal disease research laboratory (VDRL), blood urea electrolytes, creatinine, urinalysis or skin biopsy were performed on the patients.

The results they obtained showed that there were 547 (58.7%) patients utilizing depigmenting agents who met the criteria for the study, out of the 931 consecutive new patients recruited for the study. Of these, 414 (75.7%) were females and 133 (24.3%) were males within age range of 18–71 years. Traders (22.7%) accounted for the most affected, followed by businessmen and women. The duration of such practice varied from 3 months to 30 years. Utilization of topical steroid amounted to 57.2% (313) patients for depigmenting cosmetic agents. 5.9% (32) of participants agreed they were utilizing them as medication for various skin or surface body conditions such as eczema, papulosquamous disorders, sycosis barbae and connective tissue disorders. More than 21 different steroid-containing products were utilized, mostly class 1 steroid in 89.6% cases. These products include Topifram®, Topicort®, Topgel®, Topsyn®, Movate®, Dermovate®, Diprosone®, Visible Difference®, Betadine®, Bio Claire®, Betnovate–N, Neomedol®, Synalar®, Locacorten®, Palmer's Spot Remover®, Top Clear Skin®, Betnovate–C®, Neutone®, etc. Skin disorders documented during dermatologic/systemic examination included widespread dermatophyte infections with lesions, and diagnosis was frequently delayed or missed (tinea incognito). The distribution among the participants were, on the body in 191 (34.9%), macular hyper pigmentation of the face accounted for 204 (37.3%) cases, and these caused observable inflamed pustules and micropapular eruption masking the entire face. Pityriasis versicolor was very noticeable and situated at unusual sites, like the medial aspect of the upper and lower limbs among 31 (5.7%) patients. They had deep depigmentation and are linked with superficial atrophy; three patients among them had been associated with diabetes mellitus which is in early stage. Other disorders and complications observed were widespread striae in 161 (28.3%) cases, telangiectasia in 117 (21.3%), easy bruisability in 95 (17.4%) and hypertrichosis in 73 (13.3%) cases. The study concluded that cosmetic use of topical steroids exposes the users to several cutaneous complications alongside medical and aesthetic problems.

Amit et al. [33] determined lead and cadmium in cosmetic products, like soap, face cream, shampoo and shaving creams, using atomic absorption spectrophotometer. In samples consisting of a total of three different brands (coded A–C) of each product and total five samples of one brand of each sample collected from various retail shops from local market of Gwalior, India, the highest concentration of lead was detected in soap with brand code B (1.59 mg $g^{-1}$), while face cream, brand code C (0.07 mg $g^{-1}$) and talcum powder and brand codes B and C (0.24 and 0.25 mg $g^{-1}$) showed lowest lead content. For comparison between same products with different brands, mostly brand A showed the highest concentration (soap, 4.63 mg $g^{-1}$; face cream, 0.03 mg $g^{-1}$; shampoo, 1.49 mg $g^{-1}$; shaving cream, 0.69 mg $g^{-1}$; and talcum powder, 0.38 mg $g^{-1}$) followed by brand B (soap, 4; face cream, 0.05; shampoo, 1.59 mg $g^{-1}$; shaving cream, 0.66 mg $g^{-1}$; and talcum powder, 0.25 mg $g^{-1}$). The highest concentration of cadmium was detected in shampoo with brand code A (0.042 mg $g^{-1}$) followed by soap with A and B brand (0.04 and 0.037 mg $g^{-1}$). The findings showed that lead is a major toxic heavy metal in cosmetic products.

Oyelakin et al. [34] assessed the level of mercury in soaps by the use of cold vapour fluorescence spectrophotometric analysis in Gambia; a total of 16 brands of soaps were analysed. These brands of soap were grouped under four categories: medicated, toilet, skin lightening and laundry soaps. The soaps, purchased from different supermarkets in the Gambia, were used for analyses. They showed that all 16 soap brands contained mercury with concentration ranging from 2.87ng/g to 12.61 ng/g.

The World Health Organization [6] review on mercury in skin lightening products revealed that mercury is a common ingredient found in skin lightening soaps and creams as well as other cosmetics such as eye makeup, cleaning products and mascara. It stated that skin lightening soaps and creams are more commonly used in certain Africa and Asian nations and also among dark-skinned populations in Europe and North America. It further stated that mercury salts inhibit the formation of melanin, resulting in lighter skin tone. The review showed countries of greatest cosmetic use in Africa, Mali, Senegal, South Africa, Togo and Nigeria in order of increasing usage by women as 25, 27, 35, 59 and 77% are reported to use skin lightening products on a regular basis. Close to 40% of women surveyed in China, Malaysia, the Philippines and Republic of Korea in the year 2004 were reported to have used skin lighteners, while in India, 61% of the dermatological market were made of skin lightening products. The result also showed that skin lightening products are manufactured in many countries such as the Dominican Republic, Lebanon, Mexico, Pakistan, the Philippines, Thailand and the United States, and mercury-containing skin lightening products are available for sale over the internet, while individuals from Brazil, Kyrgzstan, Mexico, and the Russian Federation believe that mercury-containing skin lightening products are easy to obtain. Furthermore, the result revealed that skin lightening products come in different forms, including soap and creams, with the soap containing approximately 1–3% mercury iodide, and the cream is composed of 1–10% mercury ammonium (some soap products tested contained mercury at concentrations of up to 31 mg/kg, whereas cream products had mercury at concentration as high as 33,000 mg/kg).

Oyedeji et al. [2] ascertained hydroquinone, chromium and aluminium levels in cosmetics are marketed in Nigeria with the aim of proving that they contained poisonous substances at levels harmful to the populace; 80 cosmetic emulsions were purchased from a wholesale supermarket in Ibadan, Southwest Nigeria. The various cosmetic emulsions country of manufacture were determined by inspection of labels on the cosmetic packaging. The concentration of hydroquinone (HQ) was determined using a UV spectrophotometer. Heavy metals in the emulsion were determined by atomic absorption spectrophotometer. The study concluded that most of the cosmetic emulsion did not contain hydroquinone at levels that are detrimental to the skin, while the heavy metals were within acceptable values.

Nduka et al. [35, 36] assessed the cancer and no cancer risk of heavy metals, steroids, hydroquinone, nitrosamines and nitrites in 42 cosmetic brands purchased from cosmetic shops in Southeastern Nigeria through dermal exposure pathway; the total cancer risk value for both the cosmetic products manufactured in Nigeria and the cosmetic products manufactured outside Nigeria was less than the regulatory purpose acceptable or tolerable risk level of $10^{-6}$ to $10^{-4}$ set by USEPA [37]. This implies that the low levels of these carcinogenic elements to which users of these cosmetics are continually exposed to through the dermal exposure pathway alone over their lifetime are unlikely to pose a non-cancer and cancer risk. This therefore confers a measure of safety and no toxicological concern, but the values for total cancer risk and non-cancer risk subsist entirely on the risk contributed by the heavy metals and do not contain any risk that may be contributed by other hazardous substances as well as from other more common exposure pathways such as inhalation and ingestion.

## 6. Toxicological effect of harmful substances in cosmetics

Minimal exposure level to arsenic can lead to serious illness or death [38]. Result from Chile establishes a dose-dependent relation between chronic arsenic exposure and various forms of cancer, especially when other risk factors, such as cigarette smoking, are joined. The effect is established to persist below 50 ppb of arsenic [39]. Studies on inorganic arsenic exposure suggest a small but measurable risk increase for bladder cancer at 10 ppb [40]. The acute poisoning effects of cadmium are nausea, vomiting, diarrhoea, headache and shock; inhalation of its dust and fumes can cause cough, respiratory distress, congestion of lungs and broncho-pneumonia [41]. The metal accumulates in the liver and kidneys, damaging these organs when the exposure is chronic. Biological half-life of cadmium in humans is estimated at 20–30 years. Cadmium is listed by the United States Environmental Protection Agency [42] as one of the priority pollutant metal [43]. Absorption of lead into the skin is governed by chemical structure; therefore, skin organic lead absorption into the body tissues is more rapid than with inorganic lead compounds because of greater lipid solubility; large amounts of lead gain access to nerve tissue [44]. Acute effects of lead intake are ataxia, headache, vomiting, stupor, hallucination, tremors and convulsions. Chronic cases include weight loss, anaemia, kidney damage and memory loss. Lead bioaccumulates in bones and teeth, and it is classified as an environmental priority pollutant by the US EPA. The safe level for drinking water is 15 μg/L [41].

Skin contact with nickel can cause dermatitis, and a type of chronic eczema known as 'nickel itch' is caused by hypersensitivity reactions of nickel on the skin [45]. Oral toxicity of nickel is very low, but ingestion results to hyperglycerine and depression of the central nervous system. Large dose inhalation of nickel dust can cause lung and sinus cancer in humans. Nickel and certain of its compounds are listed by International Agency for Research on Cancer (IARC) under group 2B carcinogens as possibly carcinogenic to humans [45].

$Cr^{6+}$ is regarded as cancer-causing agent and is toxic [17]. It is corrosive to skin and causes denaturation and precipitation of tissue proteins. Chronic exposure may lead to cancer of the respiratory tract [17] and should be controlled in such a manner that no person is exposed to carcinogenic chromium (VI) at concentrations greater than 25 mg/m$^3$ of air, determined as the time-weighted average (TWA) concentration limit for up to a 10-hour workday or a 40-hr work week, over a working lifetime [44]. Chronic inhalation of manganese dust or fumes can cause manganism, a nonfatal disease which affects the central nervous system. The symptoms are mental disorder and disturbance in speech [45].

Mercury can cause both chronic and acute poisoning. Case control studies have shown effects such as tremors, impaired cognitive skills and sleep disturbance in workers with chronic exposure to mercury vapour even at low concentrations in the range 0.7–42 μg/m$^3$ [46, 47]. A study has shown that acute exposure (4–8 hours) to calculated elemental mercury levels of 1.1–44 mg/m$^3$ resulted in chest pain, dyspnoea, cough, haemoptysis, impairment of pulmonary function and evidence of interstitial pneumonitis [48]. Occupational exposure has resulted in broad-ranging functional disturbance, including erythrism, irritability, excitability, excessive shyness and insomnia. In regular and consistent use, a fine tremor develops and may escalate to violent muscular spasms. Long-term, low-level exposure has been associated with more subtle symptoms of erythrism, including fatigue, irritability, loss of memory, vivid dreams and depression [49, 50].

In 2006, the United States Food and Drug Administration revoked the approval of the use of hydroquinone and proposed a ban on all over-the-counter preparations [51], because it felt that hydroquinone cannot be ruled out as a potential carcinogen. The reason was based on the absorption in humans and the incidence of neoplasm in rats shown by several studies in which adult rats showed increased rates of tumour development [51].

Extensive literature documentation reveals that hydroquinone can cause exogenous ochronosis, a disease that deposits blue-black coloration on the skin, if taken orally; but skin preparations containing the ingredient are administered topically [51, 52]. Although proper use of hydroquinone as skin lightening agent can be effective, it causes skin sensitivity. The effect can be minimized by daily use of sunscreen with a high persistent pigment darkening (PPD) rating. Hydroquinone can be combined with alpha hydroxy acids which exfoliate the skin to quicken the lightening process. In the United States, skin creams usually contain up to 2% of hydroquinone, but higher amounts up to 4% or above should be prescribed and used with caution.

The most trending research and publication shows that minor constituents of other chemicals such as phthalates, parabens and phenols in personal care products (shampoos, toothpaste, soap, etc.), though not extensively discussed, can cause early puberty in young girls and boys. The chemicals can enter the body by cutaneous penetration through the skin, inhalation or accidental ingestion. A worrisome aspect is that exposure is very much possible through mothers during pregnancy and breastfeeding [53].

### 6.1 Skin depigmentation

In human medicine, hydroquinone is used as a topical application in skin whitening to reduce the colour of skin by decreasing the production of melanin pigment in the skin. Since hydroquinone lightens the skin by reducing melanin, it simultaneously increases exposure of the skin to UV rays, thereby increasing skin cancer risks due to UV exposure [54]. It does not have the same predisposition to cause dermatitis as metals do. This use is banned in some countries, including the member states of the European Union under Directive 76/768/EEC: 1976 [55].

### 6.2 Mechanism of whitening agent

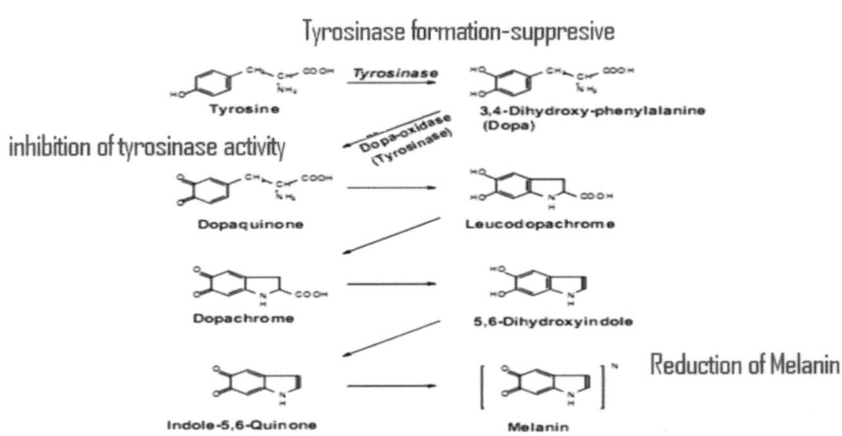


Clinical trials and experimental results prove that corticosteroids can cause permanent eye damage by inducing central serous retinopathy (CSR) or central serous chorioretinopathy (CSC) [56]. Different steroid medications, from anti-allergy nasal sprays (Nasonex, Flonase) to topical skin creams, eye drops (Tobradex) and prednisone, have been implicated in the development of CSR [57].

Corticosteroids have been applied on people with traumatic brain injury. In a systematic study in which the authors recommended that people with traumatic head injury should not be routinely treated with corticosteroids [58], side effects, such as cutaneous addiction with the development of uncomfortable and unsightly dermatoses, can occur with just one 15 g tube of moderate steroid over a period of 1 year [59].

The use of corticosteroids have severe side effects such as steroid psychosis [60], hyperglycaemia, insulin resistance, diabetes mellitus, osteoporosis, cataract, anxiety, depression, colitis, hypertension, ictus, erectile dysfunction, hypogonadism, hypothyroidism, amenorrhoea and retinopathy [61]. Evidence for corticosteroids causing peptic ulceration is relatively poor except for high doses taken for over a month [62]; majority of doctors as of 2010 still believe this is the case and would consider protective prophylactic measures [63]. Corticosteroids have a low but significant teratogenic effect, causing a few birth defects per 1000 pregnant women treated. Corticosteroids are therefore contraindicated in pregnancy [64].

Nitrosamine has been established to cause cancer in animal species, which suggests that it may also be carcinogenic in humans. Available prove from case-control studies on nitrite and nitrosamine intake implicates it in gastric cancer (GC) risk and oesophageal cancer (OC) [28].

According to Lautenschläger [27], there is no hard evidence on carcinogenic effect of nitrosamine-contaminated products applied on the skin. The study suggests that it is limited to nitrosamines inhaled with cigarette smoke or those formed by sodium nitrite from nitrite cured food reacting with secondary amines from vegetables or other food components. The study stated that although there is no 100% protection, as secondary amines and nitrite also occur in the natural environment, however, as far as cosmetic products are concerned, it should be taken care that nitrosamines and their co-chemicals such as secondary amines and nitrites are not used in the formulation. It may be a fact that health risk involved with contaminated surface body care products may be ignored as they are not supposed to remain on the skin. Also, consumers can now hive a sign of relief by drawing attention to the fact that the human system is equipped with its own secondary amines; therefore the skin can fight off any so as to protect itself with its natural moisturizing factor (NMF) which mainly contains amino acids. Chemical constituents of these amino acids are regarded as primary amines that can interact with $NO_2$, but when the molecule is destroyed in the process, nonhazardous nitrogen is normally formed.

Nitrite is approximately 10 times more toxic than nitrate [65], and interaction of nitrite with haemoglobin occurs in the blood as methaemoglobin is formed; this compound drastically lowers oxygen carrying capacity of the blood; when this happens, it results to methaemoglobinemia or 'blue baby syndrome' in infants; this is caused by lack of acidity condition in the intestinal walls of infants that is supposed to kill or reduce the bacteria; as a result these bacteria convert nitrate into nitrite. The most outstanding symptom of methaemoglobinemia is the appearance of a bluish colouration on the skin around the eyes and mouth as evidence of shortage of blood. The medical condition is treatable on early detection using methylene blue injection, which changes methaemoglobin back to haemoglobin, but death is sure when over 70% of the body's haemoglobin has been replaced by methaemoglobin [29].

Exposure to heat can cause damage to any cosmetic or makeup products. It changes the chemical formula, evaporates water and separates oil composition from other ingredients (an occurrence referred to as creaming) [66]. It also encourages the emergence of a culture medium for bacteria. The effect of these changes on the skin is harmful as such cosmetic product would no longer satisfy its optimal role [67].

## 7. Conclusions

We conclude that apart from mercury, steroids and hydroquinone, a variety of other poisonous chemicals which are prohibited by many country's regulatory authorities are still present in many cosmetics. In many cases, cosmetic product manufacturers, importers and marketers conceal the real constituent of cosmetics by not listing them in the product label. Cosmetic and skin lightening products are in high usage in every country of the world, especially among women of all ages, even with the knowledge of hazardous effect it possess to human health. Skin rashes, multiple stretch marks, yellowish brown colouration, hypertension, diabetes mellitus, renal failure and cancer are some of the toxicological and health hazards associated with cosmetic product usage and are linked to poisonous substances used in cosmetic preparation.


## Author details

John Kanayochukwu Nduka[1*], Henrietta Ijeoma Kelle[2] and Isaac Omoche Odiba[3]

1 Environmental Chemistry and Toxicology Research Unit, Pure and Industrial Chemistry Department, Nnamdi Azikiwe University, Awka, Nigeria

2 Department of Pure and Applied Science, Faculty of Sciences, National Open University, Abuja, Nigeria

3 Department of Chemistry, Alvan Ikoku Federal College of Education, Owerri, Nigeria

*Address all correspondence to: johnnduka2000@yahoo.co.uk

## References

[1] Adepoju-Bello AA, Oguntibeju OO, Adebishi RA, Okpala N, Coker HAB. Evaluation of the concentration of toxic metals in cosmetic products in Nigeria. African Journal of Biotechnology. 2012;**11**(97):16360-16364

[2] Oyedeji FO, Hassan GO, Adeleke BB. Hydroquinone and heavy metal levels in cosmetics marketed in Nigeria. Trends in Applied Science Research. 2011;**6**:622-639

[3] Hill JW. Chemistry for Changing Times. 6th ed. New York: Macmillan Company; 1992. pp. 610-615

[4] Odumosu PO, Ekwe TO. Identification and spectrometric determination of hydroquinone levels in some cosmetic creams. African Journal of Pharmacy and Pharmacology. 2010;**4**(5):231-234

[5] Scientific Committee on Consumer Safety (SCCS). Opinion on Nitosamines and Secondary Amines in Cosmetic Products. 27 March 2012

[6] WHO. Mercury in Skin Lightening Products. Geneva: World Health Organization; 2011. Available from: http://www.who.int/ipcs/assessment/public_health/mercury/en /index.html [Retrieved: 10-10-2013]

[7] Adebajo SB. An epidemiological survey of the use of cosmetic skin lightening cosmetics among traders in Lagos, Nigeria. West African Journal of Medicine. 2002;**21**(1):51-55

[8] Nnorom IC, Igwe JC, Oji-Nnorom CG. Trace metal contents of facial (make-up) cosmetics commonly used in Nigeria. African Journal of Biotechnology. 2005;**4**:1133-1138

[9] Nnoruka E, Okoye O. Topical steroid abuse: Its use as a dipigmenting agent. Journal of National Medical Association. 2006;**98**:934-939

[10] Nigeria Nursing World. Alert notice on banned products. 2012. Available from: http://www.nursingworldnigeria.com/.../nafdac-alert-notice-on-banned-products [Retrieved: 10-10-2013]

[11] National Literacy Survey. The National Literacy Survey. 2010. Available from: http://www.nigeriastat.gov.ng/pages/download/43. [Retrieved: 15-09-2013]

[12] Apaolaza-Ibanez V, Hartmann P, Deihi S, Terlutter R. Women satisfaction with cosmetic brands: The role of dissatisfaction and hedonic brand benefits. African Journal of Business Management. 2011;**5**(3):792-802

[13] Briganti S, Camera E, Picardo M. Chemical and instrumental approaches to treat hyperpigmentation. Pigment Cell & Melanoma Research. 2003;**16**:101-110

[14] Environmental Defence. Heavy Metal Hazard—The Health Risks of Hidden Heavy Metals in Cosmetics: Toronto. 2011;**1**:3-10

[15] Lee JD. Concise Inorganic Chemistry. 5th ed. London: Blackwell Science Ltd; 1996

[16] Klassen RA, Douma SL, Ford A, Rencz A, Grunsky E. Geoscience Modeling of Relative Variation in Natural Arsenic Hazard in Potential in New Brunswick. Geological Survey of Canada; 2009 [Retrieved: October 14, 2012]

[17] Patnaik P. A Handbook of Inorganic Chemicals. 1st ed. New York: McGraw Hill Publishers; 2003. pp. 140-609

[18] Lide DR. CRC Handbook of Chemistry and Physics (86th ed). Boca Raton, FL: CRC Press; 2005. pp. 4.125-4.126. ISBN: 0-8493-0486-5

[19] Norrby LJ. Why is mercury liquid? Or, why do relativistic effects not get

into chemistry textbooks. Journal of Chemical Education. 1991;**68**(2):110. DOI: 10.1021/ed068p110 [Retrieved: 10-10-2013]

[20] Senese F. Why is mercury a liquid at STP? General Chemistry Online at Frostburg State University; 2007 [Retrieved: 10-10-2013]

[21] Surmann P, Zeyat H. Voltammetric analysis using a self-renewable non-mercury electrode. Analytical and Bioanalytical Chemistry. 2005;**383**(6):1009-1013. DOI: 10.1007/s00216-005-0069-7

[22] FDA. Thimerosal in Vaccines. Center for Biologics Evaluation and Research, U.S. Food and Drug Administration. 2007 [Retrieved: 10-10-2013]

[23] Liu J, Shi JZ, Yu LM, Goyer RA, Waalkes MP. Mercury in traditional medicines: Is cinnabar toxicologically similar to common mercurials? Experimental Biology and Medicine (Maywood). 2008;**233**(7):810-817. DOI: 10.3181/0712-MR-336

[24] CIDPUSA. Mercury in your eye. 2008. Available at: http://www.cidpusa.org/mercury.htm [Retrieved: 10-10-2013]

[25] McKelvey W, Jeffery N, Clark N, Kass D, Parsons PJ. Population-based inorganic mercury biomonitoring and the identification of skin care products as a source of exposure in New York City. Environmental Health Perspective. 2011;**119**(2):203-209. DOI: 10.1289/ehp.1002396

[26] Oxford University. Safety Data for Mercuric Sulphide. Oxford University; 2009 [Retrieved: 2009-07-07]

[27] Lautenschläger H. Nitrosamines in cosmetic products—Risk of skin problems. Kosmetische Praxis. 2006;**2**:12-14

[28] Jakszyn P, Gonzalez CA. Nitrosamine and related food intake and gastric and oesophageal cancer risk: A systematic review of the epidemiological evidence. World Journal of Gastroenterology. 2006;**12**(27):4296-4303

[29] Genentech. Hazardous Substances. 2014. Available from: http://www.lenntech.com/hazardous substances/nitrite.htm [Retrieved: 06-12-2014]

[30] Phillip MH. Ullmann's Encyclopedia of Industrial Chemistry. Weinheim: Wiley-VCH; 2002, 2005. DOI: 10.1002/14356007.a13_499

[31] Moss GP. Nomenclature of steroids (recommendations 1989). Pure & Applied Chemistry. 1989;**61**(10): 1783-1822. DOI: 10.1351/pac198961101783. [Retrieved: 10-10-2013]

[32] International Union of Biochemistry and Molecular Biology. Lanosterol biosynthesis. In: Recommendations on Biochemical & Organic Nomenclature, Symbols & Terminology. 1989

[33] Amit SC, Rekha B, Atul KS, Sharad SL, Dinesh KC, Vinayak ST. Determination of lead and cadmium in cosmetic products. Journal of Chemical and Pharmaceutical Research. 2010;**2**(6):92-97

[34] Oyelakin O, Saidykhan J, Secka P, Adjivon A, Acquaye HB. Assessment of the level of mercury present in soaps by the use of cold vapour fluorescence spectrometric analysis—A Gambian case study. Ethiopian Journal of Environmental Studies and Management. 2010;**3**(1):8-12

[35] Nduka JK, Odiba IO, Aghoghome EI, Umedum LN, Nwosu MJ. Evaluation of harmful substances and health risk assessment of mercury and arsenic in cosmetic brands in Nigeria. International Journal of Chemistry. 2016;**8**(1):178-187. DOI: 10.5539/ijc.v8n1p178

[36] Nduka JK, Odiba IO, Orisakwe OE, Ukaegbu LD, Sokaibe C, Udowelle NA. Human health risk assessment of heavy metals in cosmetics in Nigeria. Journal of Cosmetic Science. 2015;**66**(4):233-246

[37] US EPA. Section 2.4.1.1, pp. 51589-51590 of the HRS rule. 2011. Available from: http://www.epa.gov/superfund/training/hrstrain/htmain/s2411.htm [Retrieved: 08-10-2014]

[38] Kozul CD, Ely KH, Enelow RI, Hamilton JW. Low dose arsenic compromises the immune response to influenza A infection in vivo. Environmental Health Perspectives. 2009;**117**(9):1441-1447. DOI: 10.1289/ehp.0900911

[39] Ferreccio C, Sancha AM. Arsenic exposure and its impact on health in Chile. Journal of Health and Population Nutrition. 2006;**24**(2):164-175

[40] Chu HA, Crawford-Brown DJ. Inorganic arsenic in drinking water and bladder cancer: A meta-analysis for dose-response assessment. International Journal of Environmental Research and Public Health. 2006;**3**(4):316-322. DOI: 10.3390/ijerph2006030039

[41] Patnaik P. A Comprehensive Guide to the Harzadous Properties of Chemical Substances. 2nd ed. New York: John Wiley and Sons; 1999. pp. 56-60

[42] Environmental Protection Agency (EPA). Health Assessment Document for Chromium. Vol. 60. Washington, USA: Environmental Protection Agency; 1984. pp. 301-305

[43] Manahan S. Toxicological Chemistry. 1st ed. Chelsea, Michigan: Lewis Publishers; 1989. pp. 43-48

[44] Sharma JL, Garg NK, Buldini PL. Condensed Chemical Dictionary. 1st ed. New Delhi: CBS Publishers; 2002

[45] International Agency for Research on Cancer (IARC). IARC Monograph 49. Geneva; 1990. pp. 3-7

[46] Liang YX, Sun RK, Sun Y, Chen ZQ, Li LH. Psychological effects of low exposure to mercury vapour: Application of computer-administered neurobehavioral evaluation system. Environmental Research. 1993;**60**(2):320-327. DOI: 10.1006/enrs.1993.1040

[47] Ngim CH, Foo SC, Boey KW, Keyaratnam J. Chronic neurobehavioral effects of elemental mercury in dentists. British Journal of Industrial Medicine. 1992;**49**(11):782-790

[48] McFarland RB, Reigel H. Chronic mercury poisoning from a single brief exposure. Journal of Occupational and Environmental Medicine. 1978;**20**(8):532. DOI: 10.1097/00043764-197808000- 00003

[49] Friberg L. Inorganic Mercury, Environmental Health Criteria 118. Geneva: World Health Organization; 1991. ISBN: 92-4-157118-7

[50] WHO. Environmental Health Criteria 1: Mercury. Geneva: World Health Organization; 1976. ISBN: 92-4-154061-3

[51] United States Food and Drug Administration (US FDA). Skin Bleaching Drug Products for Over-the-Counter Product Use. Proposed Rule (Report). 2006. 1978N-0065

[52] Olumide YM, Akinkugbe AO, Altraide D, Mohammed T, Ahamefule N, Ayanlowo S, et al. Complications of chronic use of skin lightening cosmetics. International Journal of Dermatology. 2008;**47**(4):344-353. DOI: 10.1111/j.1365-4632.2008.02719.x

[53] Harley KG, Berger KP, Kogut K, Parra K, Lustig RH, Greenspan LC, et al. Association of phthalates, parabens and

phenols found in personal care products with pubertal timing in girls and boys. Journal of Human Reproduction. 2019;**34**(1):109-117

[54] Jimbow K, Obata H, Pathak MA, Fitzpatrick TB. Mechanisms of depigmentation by hydroquinone. Journal of Investigative Dermatology. 1974;**62**:436-449

[55] EEC. Council Directive 76/768/EEC of 27 July 1976 on the approximation of the laws of the Member States relating to cosmetic products. 1976. Available from: http://eurlex.europa.eu/LexUriServ/LexUriServ.do?uri=CELEX:31976L07 68: EN: HTML. Example of a product recall in Ireland. [Retrieved: 10-10-2013]

[56] Shamsiah NS. Determination of hydroquinone and arbutin in whitening cosmetic skin care by using high performance liquid chromatography (HPLC). Malaysian Journal of Public Health Physicians' Association. 2011;**11**(4):18

[57] Carvalho-Recchia CA, Yannuzzi LA, Negrão S, Spaide RF, Freund KB, Rodriguez-Coleman H, et al. Corticosteroids and central serous chorioretinopathy. Ophthalmology. 2002;**109**(10):1834-1837. DOI: 10.1016/S0161-6420(02)01117-X

[58] Alderson P, Roberts I. Corticosteroids for acute traumatic brain injury. Cochrane Database of Systematic Reviews. 2005. DOI: 10.1002/14651858.CD000196.pub2

[59] Kenneth PF, David JE. Tortured tube sign. Western Journal of Medicine. 2001;**174**(6):383-384. DOI: 10.1136/ewjm.174.6.383

[60] Hall R. Psychiatric Adverse Drug Reactions: Steroid Psychosis. Massachusetts: Director of Research Monarch Health Corporation Marblehead; 2002

[61] Donihi AC, Raval D, Saul M, Korytkowski MT, DeVita MA. Prevalence and predictors of corticosteroid-related hyperglycemia in hospitalized patients. Endocrine Practice. 2006;**12**(4):358-362

[62] Pecora PG, Kaplan B. Corticosteroids and ulcers: Is there an association? Annals of Pharmacotherapy. 1996;**30**(7-8):870-872

[63] Martínek J, Hlavova K, Zavada F. A surviving myth—Corticosteroids are still considered ulcerogenic by a majority of physicians. Scandinavian Journal of Gastroenterology. 2010;**45**(10):1156-1161. DOI: 10.3109/00365521.2010.497935

[64] Shepard TH, Brent RL, Friedman JM, Jones KL, Miller RK, Moore CA, et al. Update on new developments in the study of human teratogens. Teratology. 2002;**65**(4):153-161. DOI: 10.1002/tera.10032

[65] Schneider NR. Overview of Nitrate and Nitrite Poisoning. 2012. Available from: http://www.merckmanuals.com/vet/toxicology/nitrate_and_nitrite_poisoning/overview_of_nitrate_and_nitrite_poisoning.html [Retrieved: 06-12-2014]

[66] Lautenschläger H. Shelf Life and Preservation. Leichlingen: Kosmetik Konzept KOKO GmbH & Co. KG; 2007. Available from: www.dermaviduals.de [Retrieved: 11-11-2014]

[67] Ioana C. How to Properly Store Cosmetics. 2010. Available from: www.metrolic.com/how-to properly-store-cosmetics-100056/ [Retrieved: 10-10-2013]

Chapter 5

# Mechanism and Health Effects of Heavy Metal Toxicity in Humans

*Godwill Azeh Engwa, Paschaline Udoka Ferdinand, Friday Nweke Nwalo and Marian N. Unachukwu*

## Abstract

Several heavy metals are found naturally in the earth crust and are exploited for various industrial and economic purposes. Among these heavy metals, a few have direct or indirect impact on the human body. Some of these heavy metals such as copper, cobalt, iron, nickel, magnesium, molybdenum, chromium, selenium, manganese and zinc have functional roles which are essential for various diverse physiological and biochemical activities in the body. However, some of these heavy metals in high doses can be harmful to the body while others such as cadmium, mercury, lead, chromium, silver, and arsenic in minute quantities have delirious effects in the body causing acute and chronic toxicities in humans. The focus of this chapter is to describe the various mechanism of intoxication of some selected heavy metals in humans along with their health effects. Therefore it aims to highlight on biochemical mechanisms of heavy metal intoxication which involves binding to proteins and enzymes, altering their activity and causing damage. More so, the mechanism by which heavy metals cause neurotoxicity, generate free radical which promotes oxidative stress damaging lipids, proteins and DNA molecules and how these free radicals propagate carcinogenesis are discussed. Alongside these mechanisms, the noxious health effects of these heavy metals are discussed.

**Keywords:** heavy metals, toxicity, neurotoxicity, carcinogenesis, free radicals, health effects

## 1. Introduction

Metals are natural constituents that exist in the ecosystem. They are substances with high electrical conductivity which voluntarily lose their electrons to form cations. Metals are found all over the earth including the atmosphere, earth crust, water bodies, and can also accumulate in biological organisms including plants and animals. Among the 35 natural existing metals, 23 possess high specific density above 5 g/cm$^3$ with atomic weight greater than 40.04 and are generally termed heavy metals [1, 2]. Theses metals generally termed heavy metals include: antimony, tellurium, bismuth, tin, thallium, gold, arsenic, cerium, gallium, cadmium, chromium, cobalt, copper, iron, lead, mercury, manganese, nickel, platinum, silver, uranium, vanadium, and zinc [1, 2]. This category of metals termed heavy metals have not only been known for their high density but most importantly for their adverse effects to the ecosystem and living organisms [3]. Some of these heavy metals such as cobalt, chromium, copper, magnesium, iron, molybdenum, manganese, selenium, nickel and zinc are essential nutrients that are required for various physiological and biochemical functions in the body and may result to deficiency diseases or syndromes if not in adequate amounts [4] but in large doses they may cause acute or chronic toxicities.

These heavy metals are distributed in the environment through several natural processes such as volcanic eruptions, spring waters, erosion, and bacterial activity, and through anthropogenic activities which include fossil fuel combustion, industrial processes, agricultural activities as well as feeding [5]. These heavy metals do bioaccumulate in living organisms and the human body through various processes causing adverse effects. In the human body, these heavy metals are transported and compartmentalized into body cells and tissues binding to proteins, nucleic acids destroying these macromolecules and disrupting their cellular functions. As such, heavy metal toxicity can have several consequences in the human body. It can affect the central nervous function leading to mental disorder, damage the blood constituents and may damage the lungs, liver, kidneys and other vital organs promoting several disease conditions [6]. Also, long term accumulation of heavy metals in the body may result in slowing the progression of physical, muscular and neurological degenerative processes that mimic certain diseases such as Parkinson's disease and Alzheimer's disease [6]. More so, repeated long-term contact with some heavy metals or their compounds may even damage nucleic acids, cause mutation, mimic hormones thereby disrupting the endocrine and reproductive system and eventually lead to cancer [7].

This chapter will highlight on the various sources of heavy metals and the processes that promote their exposure and bioaccumulation in the human body. More focus will be laid on the various mechanisms that lead to heavy metal toxicity with emphasis on macromolecule and cellular damages, carcinogenesis, neurotoxicity and the molecular basis for their noxious effects. The various toxic effects along with the signs and symptoms of some heavy metals in the human body will be discussed.

## 2. Sources of heavy metal exposure to humans

Heavy metals are naturally present in our environment. They are present in the atmosphere, lithosphere, hydrosphere and biosphere [8]. Although these heavy metals are present in the ecosystem, their exposure to humans is through various anthropogenic activities of man. In the earth crust, these heavy metals are present in ores which are recovered during mining activities as minerals. In most ores heavy metals such as arsenic, iron, lead, zinc, gold, nickel, silver and cobalt exist as sulfides while others such as manganese, aluminum, selenium gold, and antimony exist as oxides. Certain heavy metals such as copper, iron and cobalt can exist both as sulfide and oxide ores. Some sulfides may contain two or more heavy metals together such as chalcopyrite, ($CuFeS_2$) which contains both copper and iron. During these mining activities, heavy metals are released from the ore and scattered in open in the environment; left in the soil, transported by air and water to other areas. Furthermore, when these heavy metals are used in the industries for various industrial purposes, some of these elements are released into the air during combustion or into the soil or water bodies as effluents. More so, the industrial products such as paints, cosmetics, pesticides, and herbicides also serve as sources of heavy metals. Heavy metals may be transported through erosion, run-off or acid rain to different locations on soils and water bodies. As reviewed from [9], the sources of specific heavy metals are described below.

### 2.1 Arsenic

Arsenic is the 20th most abundant element on earth and the 33rd on the periodic table. The inorganic forms such as arsenite and arsenate compounds are lethal to humans and other organisms in the environment. Humans get in contact with arsenic through several means which include industrial sources such as smelting and microelectronic industries. Drinking water may be contaminated with arsenic which is present in wood preservatives, herbicides, pesticides, fungicides and paints [10].

### 2.2 Lead

Lead is a slightly bluish, bright silvery metal in a dry atmosphere. The main sources of lead exposure include drinking water, food, cigarette, industrial processes and domestic sources. The industrial sources of lead include gasoline, house paint, plumbing pipes, lead bullets, storage batteries, pewter pitchers, toys and faucets [11]. Lead is released into the atmosphere from industrial processes as well as from vehicle exhausts. Therefore, it may get into the soil and flow into water bodies which can be taken up by plants and hence human exposure of lead may also be through food or drinking water [12].

### 2.3 Mercury

The metallic mercury is a shiny silver-white, odorless liquid metal which becomes colorless and odorless gas upon heating. Mercury is used in producing dental amalgams, thermometers and some batteries. Also, it can be found in some chemical, electrical-equipment, automotive, metal-processing, and building industries. Mercury can exist in a gaseous form thus it can be inhaled. Other forms of mercury contamination in humans may be through anthropogenic activities such as municipal wastewater discharges, agriculture, incineration, mining, and discharges of industrial wastewater [13].

### 2.4 Cadmium

This metal is mostly used in industries for the production of paints, pigments alloys, coatings, batteries as well as plastics. Majority of cadmium, about three-fourths is used as electrode component in producing alkaline batteries. Cadmium is emitted through industrial processes and from cadmium smelters into sewage sludge, fertilizers, and groundwater which can remain in soils and sediments for several decades and taken up by plants. Therefore, significant human exposure to cadmium can be by the ingestion of contaminated foodstuffs especially cereals, grains, fruits and leafy vegetables as well as contaminated beverages [14, 15]. Also, humans may get exposed to cadmium by inhalation through incineration of municipal waste.

### 2.5 Chromium

Chromium is a metal that is present in petroleum and coal, chromium steel, pigment oxidants, fertilizers, catalyst, oil well drilling and metal plating tanneries. Chromium is extensively used in industries such as wood preservation, electroplating, metallurgy, production of paints and pigments, chemical production, tanning, and pulp and paper production. These industries play a major role in chromium pollution with an adverse effect on biological and ecological species [16]. Following the anthropogenic activities by humans, disposal of sewage and use of fertilizers may lead to the release of chromium into the environment [16]. Therefore, these

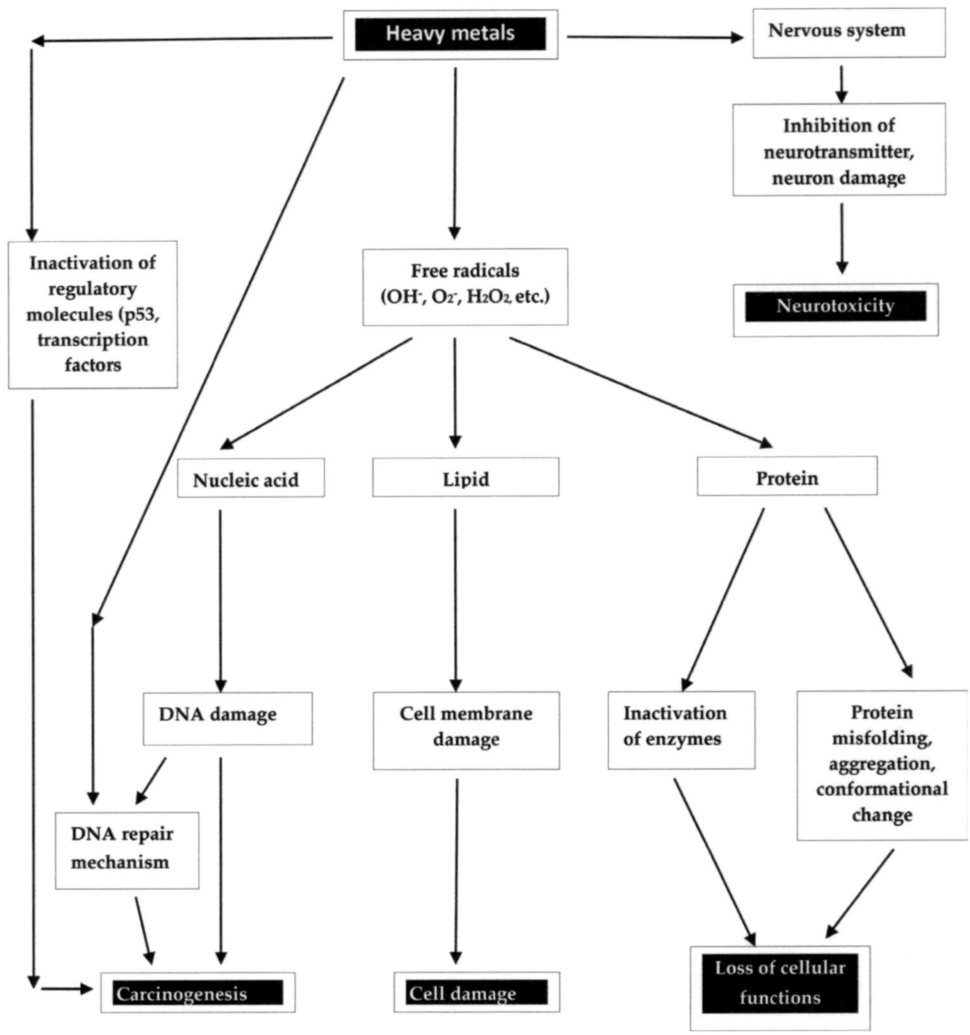


**Figure 1.**
*Pathway of heavy metals sources and exposure to humans.*

industrial and agricultural practices increase the environmental contamination of chromium. Environmental pollution by chromium has been mostly by the hexavalent chromium in recent years [17].

## 2.6 Copper

This is a heavy metal which is used in industries to produce copper pipes, cables, wires, copper cookware, etc. It is also used to make copper intrauterine devices and birth control pills. Copper in the form of copper sulfate is added to drinking water and swimming pools [18]. Due to man's anthropogenic and industrial activities, it can accumulate in the soil and up taken by plants. As such, copper is present in some nuts, avocado, wheat germ and bran etc.

## 2.7 Manganese

This metal is added to gasoline as methylcyclopentadienyl manganese tricarbonyl (MMT) and thus, gasoline fumes contain a very toxic form of manganese [19].

| Heavy metals | EPA limits in drinking water (ppm) | OSHA limit in workplace air (mg) | FDA limit in bottled water/ food (ppm) |
|---|---|---|---|
| Arsenic | 0.01 | 10 | – |
| Barium | 2.0 | 0.5 | – |
| Cadmium | 0.005 | 5 | 0.005 |
| Chromium | 0.1 | 1 | 1 |
| Lead | 0.015 | 0.15 | – |
| Mercury | 0.002 | 0.1 | 1 |
| Selenium | 0.05 | 0.2 | – |
| Silver | 0.0001 | 0.01 | – |
| Zinc | 5 | 5 | – |

*ppm, parts per million; mg, milligram; EPA, Environmental Protection Agency; OSHA, Occupational Safety and Health Administration; FDA, Food and Drug Administration.*

**Table 1.**
*Regulatory limit of selected heavy metals.*

### 2.8 Nickel

It is used in the production of batteries, nickel-plated jewelry, machine parts, nickel plating on metallic objects, manufacture of steel, cigarette smoking, wire, electrical parts, etc. Also, it can be found in food stuff such as imitation whip cream, unrefined grains and cereals, commercial peanut butter, hydrogenated vegetable oils, as well as contaminated alcoholic beverages [19]. The various sources of heavy metals are summarized in **Figure 1**.

## 3. Route of exposure, bio-uptake and bioaccumulation of heavy metals in humans

Humans may directly get in contact with heavy metals by consuming contaminated food stuffs, sea animals, and drinking of water, through inhalation of polluted air as dust fumes, or through occupational exposure at workplace [20]. The contamination chain of heavy metals almost usually follows this cyclic order: from industry, to the atmosphere, soil, water and foods then human [8]. These heavy metals can be taken up through several routes. Some heavy metals such as lead, cadmium, manganese, arsenic can enter the body through the gastrointestinal route; that is, through the mouth when eating food, fruits, vegetables or drinking water or other beverages. Others can enter the body by inhalation while others such as lead can be absorbed through the skin.

Most heavy metals are distributed in the body through blood to tissues [21]. Lead is carried by red blood cells to the liver and kidney and subsequently redistributed to the teeth, bone and hair mostly as phosphate salt [20]. Cadmium initially binds to blood cells and albumin, and subsequently binds to metallothionein in kidney and liver tissue. Following its distribution from blood to the lungs, manganese vapor diffuses across the lung membrane to the Central nervous system (CNS). Organic salts of manganese which are lipid soluble are distributed in the intestine for fecal elimination while inorganic manganese salts which are water soluble are distributed in plasma and kidney for renal elimination. Arsenic is distributed in blood and accumulates in heart, lung, liver, kidney, muscle and neural tissues and also in the skin, nails and hair. The regulatory limit for some selected heavy metals is shown in **Table 1**.

# 4. Mechanism of heavy metal toxicity

## 4.1 Heavy metal-induced oxidative stress and oxidation of biological molecules

Certain heavy metals are known to generate free radicals which may lead to oxidative stress and cause other cellular damages (see [22] for review). The mechanism of free radical generation is specific to the type of heavy metal.

### *4.1.1 Iron*

Iron is a useful heavy metal in the human body as it is a constituent of certain biological molecules like the hemoglobin and involved in various physiological activities. However, in its free state, iron is one of the heavy metals generally known to generate hydroxyl radical ($OH^{\bullet}$) as shown below by the Fenton reaction.

$$Fe^{3+} + O_2^{-} \rightarrow Fe^{2+} + O_2 \quad (1)$$

$$Fe^{2+} + H_2O_2 \rightarrow Fe^{3+} + OH^{\bullet} + OH^{-} \text{ (Fenton reaction)} \quad (2)$$

Net reaction (Haber-Weiss reaction):

$$O_2^{-} + H_2O_2 \rightarrow OH^{-} + OH^{\bullet} + O_2 \quad (3)$$

In addition to the above reactions, the following reactions below can also occur:

$$OH^{\bullet}\ H_2O_2 \rightarrow H_2O + H^{+} + O^{2\bullet-} \quad (4)$$

$$OH^{\bullet} + Fe^{2+} \rightarrow Fe^{3+} + OH^{-} \quad (5)$$

$$LOOH + Fe^{2+} \rightarrow Fe^{3+} + LO^{-} + OH^{\bullet} \quad (6)$$

Hydroxyl radical ($OH^{\bullet}$) is the most common free radical generated by the oxidation of iron. $OH^{\bullet}$ is capable of reacting with biological molecules such as proteins, lipids and DNA damaging them. When $OH^{\bullet}$ reacts with guanine, a nitrogenous base of nucleic acids, it leads to the generation of 8-oxo-7,8-dihydro-20-deoxyguanosine (8-oxo-dG) and 2,6-diamino-5-formamido-4-hydroxypyrimidine (FAPy-G), in which the former is a good marker for oxidative damage [23].

It is well documented that metal-induced generation of oxygen reactive species can attack polyunsaturated fatty acid such as phospholipids. The first of such observation was first presented by Bucher et al. [24] who showed that iron-generated $OH^{\bullet}$ can oxidize lipid membranes through a process known as lipid peroxidation. Following his experimental observations, he proposed the following mechanism:

Steps of lipid peroxidation:

$$\text{Initiation: Lipid} + R\bullet/OH^{\bullet} \rightarrow \text{Lipid}^{\bullet} \quad (7)$$

$$\text{Propagation: Lipid}^{\bullet} + O_2 \rightarrow \text{Lipid} - OO^{\bullet} \quad (8)$$

$$\text{Lipid} - \text{OO} + \text{Lipid}^{\bullet} \rightarrow \text{Lipid} - \text{OOH} + \text{Lipid}^{\bullet} \tag{9}$$

$$\text{Termination: Lipid}^{\bullet} + \text{Lipid}\bullet \rightarrow \text{Lipid} - \text{Lipid} \tag{10}$$

$$\text{Lipid} - \text{OO}\bullet + \text{Lipid}^{\bullet} \rightarrow \text{Lipid} - \text{OO} - \text{Lipid} \tag{11}$$

At the initiation stage, the radical $(R^{\bullet})/OH^{\bullet}$ attacks the lipid membrane to form a radial lipid. This radical lipid further propagates the formation of peroxyl lipid radical by reacting with dioxygen molecule or with a lipid. This reaction further promotes damage of the lipid molecule. At the termination stage, two radical lipid molecules and/or with a peroxyl lipid radical reacts to form a stable lipid molecule. The major aldehyde product of lipid peroxidation is malondialdehyde and it serves as a marker for lipid peroxidation.

Generally, proteins are not easily damaged by $H_2O_2$ and other simple oxidants unless transition metals are present. Thus, protein damaged are usually metal-catalyzed and involves oxidative scission, bityrosine cross links, loss of histidine residues, the introduction of carbonyl groups, and the formation of protein-centered alkyl (R•), alkoxyl (RO•) and alkylperoxyl (ROO•) radicals [25].

### *4.1.2 Copper*

Copper ions have been identified to participate in the formation of reactive oxygen species (ROS) as cupric ($Cu^{2+}$) and cuprous ($Cu^{1+}$) which can participate in oxidation and reduction reactions. The $Cu^{2+}$ in the presence of biological reductants such as glutathione (GSH) or ascorbic acid can be reduced to $Cu^{+}$ which is capable of catalyzing the decomposition of $H_2O_2$ to form OH• *via* the Fenton reaction [26] as shown below.

$$Cu^{+} + H_2O_2 \rightarrow Cu^{2+} + OH^{\bullet} + OH^{-} \tag{12}$$

The OH• radical formed is capable of reacting with several biomolecules. Experimental studies confirmed that copper is also capable of inducing DNA strand breaks and oxidation of bases *via* oxygen free radicals [27]. Though *in vivo* studies have not revealed copper-induced oxidation of low density lipoprotein (LDL), *in vitro* studies clearly demonstrated LDL oxidation induced by copper [28].

### *4.1.3 Chromium*

Chromium (Cr), particularly $Cr^{4+}$ has been shown in *in vitro* studies to generate free radicals from $H_2O_2$ [29]. Also, *in vivo* studies were able to show the detection of free radicals due to chromium in the liver and blood of animals. It was observed that $Cr^{5+}$ intermediates were generated as a result of one-electron reduction.

### *4.1.4 Cobalt*

Cobalt (Co), particularly $Co^{2+}$ has been shown to generate superoxide ($^{\bullet}O_2^{-}$) from the decomposition of $H_2O_2$ [30].

$$Co^{2+} + O_2 \rightarrow Co^{+} + O_2^{\bullet -} \rightarrow Co^{+} - OO\bullet \tag{13}$$

*4.1.5 Vanadium*

Vanadium is a heavy metal that occurs in various oxidative states and has been shown to generate free radical. In the plasma, vanadium (V) is rapidly reduced to vanadium (IV) by NADPH and ascorbic acid antioxidants which bind to plasma proteins for transportation [31].

$$V^{5+} + NADPH \rightarrow V^{4+} + NADP^{+} + H^{+} \quad (14)$$

$$V^{4+} + O_2 \rightarrow V^{5+} + O^{2\bullet-} \quad (15)$$

$$V^{5+} + O_2^{\bullet-} \rightarrow [V^{5+} - OO^{\bullet}] \quad (16)$$

More so under physiological conditions at approximately pH of 7, V(IV) can generate $OH^{\bullet}$ from the decomposition of $H_2O_2$ according to the Fenton reaction.

$$V^{4+} + H_2O_2 \rightarrow V^{5+} + OH^{-} + {}^{\bullet}OH \quad (17)$$

*4.1.6 Arsenic*

Arsenic has also been shown to generate free radicals such as superoxide ($O_2^{\bullet-}$), singlet oxygen ($^1O_2$), nitric oxide ($NO^{\bullet}$), hydrogen peroxide ($H_2O_2$), the peroxyl radical ($ROO^{\bullet}$) [32], dimethylarsinic peroxyl radicals ($(CH_3)_2AsOO^{\bullet}$) and also the dimethylarsinic radical ($(CH_3)_2As^{\bullet}$) [33] in some studies though the mechanism for the generation of all these reactive species remains unclear.

### 4.2 Heavy metal-induced carcinogenesis

Some heavy metals are known to have carcinogenic effect. Several signaling proteins or cellular regulatory proteins that participate in apoptosis, cell cycle regulation, DNA repair, DNA methylation, cell growth and differentiation are targets of heavy metals [34]. Thus, heavy metals may induce carcinogenic effect by targeting a number of these proteins. More so, the carcinogenic effects of certain heavy metals have been related to the activation of redox-sensitive transcription factors such as AP-1, NF-κB and p53 through the recycling of electrons by antioxidant network. These transcription factors control the expression of protective genes that induce apoptosis, arrest the proliferation of damaged cells, repair damaged DNA and power the immune system [22]. Metal signalization of transcription factor AP-1 and NF-κB has been observed in the mitogen-activated protein (MAP) kinase pathways where the nuclear transcription factor NF-κB, is involved in controlling inflammatory responses while AP-1 is involved in cell growth and differentiation [22]. The p53 protein is an important protein in cell division as it guards a cell-cycle checkpoint and control cell division [35]. Inactivation of p53 allows uncontrolled cell division and thus p53 gene disruption has been associated with most human cancers. Also, AP-1 and NF-κB family of transcription factors are involved in both cell proliferation and apoptosis, and also regulate p53. Heavy metals generated free radicals inside the cell selectively activates these transcription factors and thus, may suggest that cell proliferation or cell death may be related to the exposure to carcinogenic metals. There exist various mechanisms of heavy metal-induced carcinogenesis.

#### *4.2.1 Arsenic*

Arsenic-induced carcinogenic mechanisms include epigenetic alterations, damage to the dynamic DNA maintenance system and generation of ROS [36, 37]. Alterations of histones, DNA methylation, and miRNA are the key epigenetic changes induced by arsenic which have shown to possess potentials to cause malignant growth [37]. In vitro studies have shown arsenic to alter the expression of p53 protein which also led to decreased expression of p21, one downstream target [38]. Arsenic compounds have been shown in an *in vitro* cell line study to promote genotoxicity in humans and mice leucocytes [39]. Also, a methylated form of arsenic was shown to inhibit DNA repair processes and also generate ROS in liver and spleen as metabolic products [40]. Arsenic can bind DNA-binding proteins and disrupt the DNA repair processes thereby increasing the risk of carcinogenesis. For example, the tumor suppressor gene-coded DNA was suppressed when arsenic was bound to methyl-transferase [41]. Also, cancers of the liver, skin, prostate and Kupffer cell were associated with Arsenic poisoning.

#### *4.2.2 Lead*

The mechanism of lead-induced carcinogenic process is postulated to induce DNA damage, disrupt DNA repair system and cellular tumor regulatory genes through the generation of ROS [42]. Studies have supported with evidence that ROS generation by lead is key in altering chromosomal structure and sequence [42]. Lead can disrupt transcription processes by replacing zinc in certain regulatory proteins [42].

#### *4.2.3 Mercury*

Little is known on the potential of mercury to act as a mutagen or carcinogen. However, the proposed mechanism of mercury-induced cancer is through the generation of free radicals inducing oxidative stress thereby damaging biomolecules. Mercury has been shown to induce malignant growth through the generation of free radicals as well as disruption of DNA molecular structure, the repair and maintenance system [43].

#### *4.2.4 Nickel*

Nickel has an extensive range of carcinogenic mechanisms which include regulation of transcription factors, controlled expression of certain genes and generation of free radicals. Nickel has been shown to be implicated in regulating the expression of specific long non-coding RNAs, certain mRNAs and microRNAs. Nickel can promote methylation of promoter and induce the down regulation of maternally expressed gene 3 (MEG3) thereby upregulating hypoxia-inducible factor-1α, two proteins which are known to be implicated in carcinogenesis [44]. It has also been demonstrated that nickel can generate free radicals, which contributes to carcinogenic processes [45].

#### *4.2.5 Cadmium*

Cadmium has been implicated in promoting apoptosis, oxidative stress, DNA methylation and DNA damage.

#### *4.2.6 Iron*

The main cause of cancer due to iron intoxication is through the generation of free radicals. A school of thought produced a mechanism for iron-induced cancer whereby bile acids (deoxycholic acid), iron(II) complexes, vitamins K and oxygen interact to generate free radicals which induced oncogenic effect in the colon.

## 4.3 Heavy metal-induced neurotoxicity

Some heavy metals such as lead and manganese may affect the brain and cause neurological toxicity as reviewed from [46].

### *4.3.1 Lead*

Lead toxicity is targeted towards the memory and learning processes of the brain and can be mediated through three processes. Lead can impair learning and memory in the brain by inhibiting the N-methyl-D-aspartate receptor (NMDAR) and can block neurotransmission by inhibit neurotransmitter release, block the neuronal voltage-gated calcium ($Ca^{2+}$) channels (VGCCs) and reduce the expression of brain-derived neurotrophic factor (BDNF).

### *4.3.2 Inhibition of NMDAR*

The NMDAR is known to enhance learning and memory mediated by the hippocampus [47] as this has been confirmed in animal studies in which animals exposed to lead during its developmental process exhibit similar learning deficits comparable to those with the absence or impaired NMDARs [48, 49]. In the hippocampus, NMDAR is a neural receptor which consists of two or more subunits; an obligatory NR1 subunit and one or more subunits from the NR2 particularly NR2A, NR2B and NR3 families. Lead has been shown to be a potent, non-competitive antagonist of the NMDAR [50–53], preferentially with high affinity at a regulatory site on the NR2A subunit [54]. This has been further supported in electrophysiological studies in which recombinant receptors for the subunits have shown NR2A-NMDARs to be more potently inhibited by lead than NR2B-NMDARs [55]. More so, lead has been shown to decrease the content of NR2A in the hippocampus and also alter the expression of NR1 spliced variants [56, 57] suggesting lead exposure disrupts the normal ontogeny of NMDAR.

### *4.3.3 Reduction of neurotransmission*

Lead can decrease neurotransmission as long term exposure of rats to low levels of lead has shown reduction in the release of $Ca^{2+}$-dependent glutamate and γ-aminobutyric acid (GABA) in the hippocampus [58, 59]. This indicates dysfunction of presynaptic neuron signalization in the hippocampus as a result of lead exposure [60]. More so, lead exposure also impairs two postsynaptic currents; inhibitory post synaptic currents (IPSCs) and excitatory post synaptic currents (EPSCs) which are dependent on the release of presynaptic neurotransmitter such as glutamate and GABA. Thus, lead exposure leads to reductions in IPSCs and EPSCs indicating a deficit in glutamatergic and GABAergic neurotransmission systems. Also, lead has been shown to reduce the expression of key presynaptic proteins such as synaptobrevin (Syb) and synaptophysin (Syn) involved in vesicular neurotransmitter release [59, 60]. Lead can disrupt neurotransmission by inhibiting the neuronal voltage-gated calcium ($Ca^{2+}$) channels (VGCCs) [61]. Thus, inhibition of presynaptic VGCCs may reduce the influx of $Ca^{2+}$ which is required for fast release of vesicular neurotransmitter thus interfering with neurotransmission. It is now suggested that inhibition of either NMDARs or VGCCs by lead would result in a significant decrease of $Ca^{2+}$ influx into the cell. Reduction of $Ca^{2+}$ entry into the cell will prevent neurotransmitter release and thus impair signalization leading to neurological disease states [62, 63]. Lead can also reduce the expression of brain-derived neurotrophic factor (BDNF), a trans-synaptic signaling molecule that is released from both axons and dendrites which is involved in synaptic development and neurotransmitter release [64]. BDNF activity is also dependent on $Ca^{2+}$ and thus has been implicated in the development of neurological diseases.

#### *4.3.4 Manganese*

Manganese is known to accumulate in the mitochondria of neurons, astrocytes and oligodendrocytes cells and disrupts ATP synthesis [65] by inhibiting the F1/F0 ATP synthase [65] or complex 1 (NADH dehydrogenase) of the mitochondrial respiration chain [66]. More so, it has recently been shown that manganese inhibits ATP synthesis at two sites in the brain mitochondria which are either the glutamate/aspartate exchanger or the complex II (succinate dehydrogenase) depending on the mitochondrial energy source [67]. The disruption of ATP synthesis by manganese leads to decreased intracellular ATP levels and generation of free radicals thereby increasing oxidative stress [68] which may contribute to manganese cellular toxicity [69]. Furthermore, manganese can oxidize dopamine (DA) to react with quinone species thereby disrupting the dopaminergic system (for review, see [70]). This has been shown in animal studies were manganese exposure has led to specific deficits in the dopaminergic system [71]. The DA reactive species are taken up by the dopamine transporter (DAT1) thus causing dopaminergic neurotoxicity [72].

### 4.4 Biochemical mechanism of heavy metal toxicity

When heavy metals are ingested through food or water into the body, they are acidified by the acid medium of the stomach. In this acidic medium, they are oxidized to their various oxidative states ($Zn^{2+}$, $Cd^{2+}$, $Pb^{2+}$, $As^{2+}$, $As^{3+}$, $Ag^{+}$, $Hg^{2+}$, etc.) which can readily bind to biological molecules such as proteins and enzymes to form stable and strong bonds. The most common functional group that heavy metals bind is the thio groups (SH group of cysteine and $SCH_3$ group of methionine). Cadmium has been shown to inhibit human thiol transferases such as thioredoxin reductase, glutathione reductase, thioredoxin *in vitro* by binding to cysteine residues in their active sites [73]. The equations of these reactions are shown below (see [74] for review) (**Figure 2**).

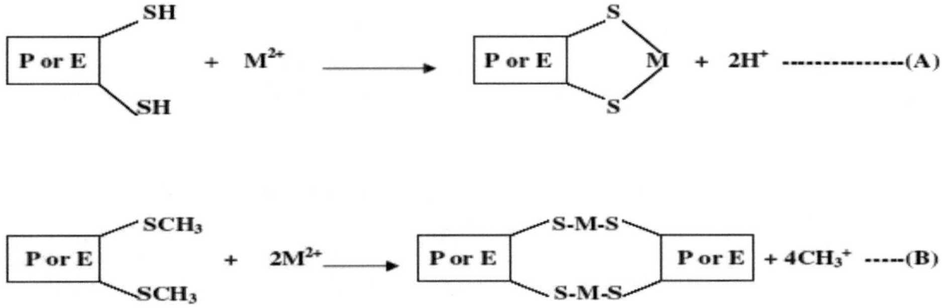


**Figure 2.**
*Reactions of Heavy metals with sulphydryl groups of proteins or enzymes (A) = Intramolecular bonding; (B) = Intermolecular bonding; P = Protein; E = Enzyme; M = Metal.*

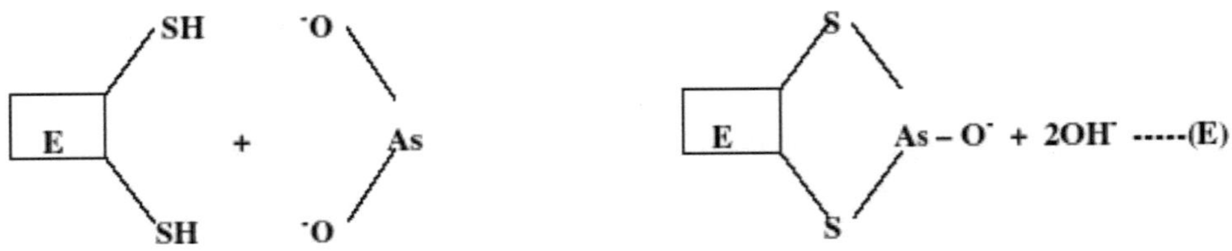


**Figure 3.**
*Reaction of arsenic with the thio group of enzymes.*

In the above reaction, the oxidized heavy metal replaces the hydrogen of the SH group and the methyl of the $SCH_3$ group thereby inhibiting the function of the protein or activity of the enzyme. For example, methylmercury (MeHg) strongly inhibits the activity of L-glutamine D-fructose-6-phosphate amidotransferase in yeast [75].

Heavy metal-bound proteins may be a substrate for certain enzymes. In such situations, the heavy metal-bound protein fits into an enzyme in a highly specific pattern to form an enzyme-substrate complex and thus cannot accommodate any other substrate until it is freed. As such, the product of the substrate is not formed as the enzyme is blocked and therefore, the heavy metal remains embedded in the tissue leading to dysfunctions, abnormalities and damages in the body. Inhibition of thiol transferases lead to increased oxidative stress and cell damage. For example, toxic arsenic present in fungicides, herbicides and insecticides can attack –SH groups in enzymes to inhibit their catalytic activities as shown in **Figure 3**.

Also, heavy metal toxicity may be induced by the replacement of a metalloenzyme by another metal ion of similar size. Cadmium displaces zinc and calcium ions from zinc finger proteins and metalloproteins [76, 77]. For instance, cadmium can replace zinc in certain dehydrogenating enzymes, leading to cadmium toxicity. Such replacement can convert the enzyme structurally to an inactive form and completely alter its activity. These heavy metals in their ionic species such as $Pb^{2+}$, $Cd^{2+}$, $Ag^{+}$ $Hg^{2+}$ and $As^{3+}$ form very stable biotoxic compounds with proteins and enzymes and are difficult to be dissociated.

Heavy metals may also inhibit protein folding. This was first observed when heavy metals such as cadmium, lead, mercury and arsenite were shown to effectively interfere with the refolding of chemically denatured proteins [78]. It was also observed that when protein misfolded in the presence of heavy metals, the misfolded protein could not be rescued in the presence of reduced glutathione or EDTA chelator. The order of heavy metal in terms of their efficacy in folding inhibition is mercury > cadmium > lead and correlates with the relative stability of their monodentate complexes with imidazole, thiol and carboxylate groups in proteins [79].

Heavy metal may cause proteins to aggregate as arsenite-induced protein aggregation was observed and shown to be concentration-dependent. Also, the aggregates contained a wide variety of proteins enriched in functions related to metabolism, protein folding, protein synthesis and stabilization [79]. *Saccharomyces cerevisiae* (budding yeast) cells was shown to accumulate aggregated proteins after it was exposed to equi-toxic concentrations of cadmium, arsenite and chromium (Cr(VI)) and the effect of protein aggregation was influenced by heavy metals in this order: arsenic > cadmium > chromium [80]. The *in vivo* potency of these agents to trigger protein aggregation probably depends on the efficiency of their cellular uptake/export and on their distinct modes of biological action. Summarized in **Figure 4** is the various mechanisms of heavy metal intoxication.

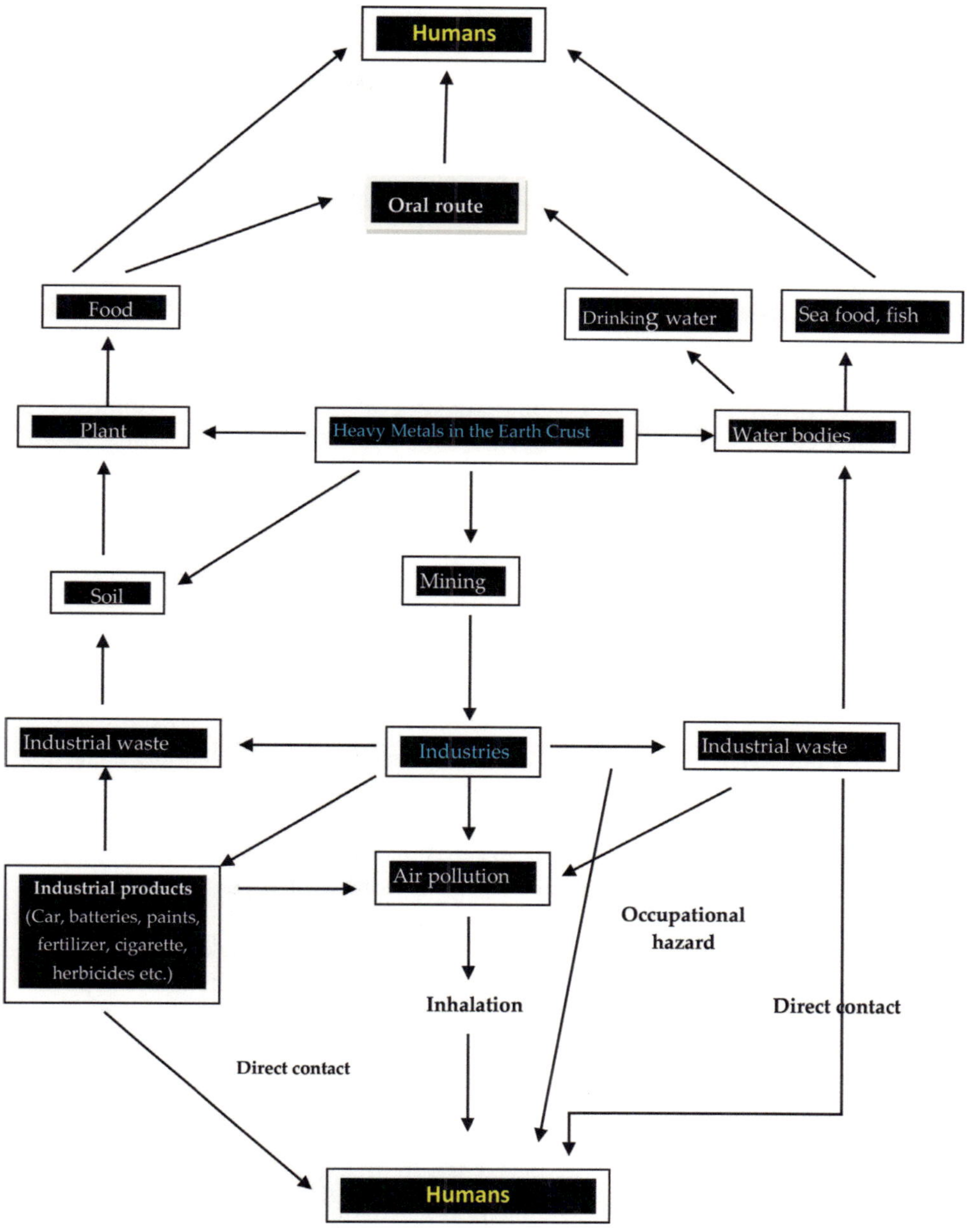


**Figure 4.**
*Mechanisms of heavy metal intoxication in humans.*

## 5. Health effects of heavy metal toxicity in humans

Heavy metal toxicity can have several health effects in the body. Heavy metals can damage and alter the functioning of organs such as the brain, kidney, lungs, liver, and blood. Heavy metal toxicity can either be acute or chronic effects. Long-term exposure of the body to heavy metal can progressively lead to muscular, physical and neurological degenerative processes that are similar to diseases such as Parkinson's disease, multiple sclerosis, muscular dystrophy and Alzheimer's disease. Also, chronic long-term exposure of some heavy metals may cause cancer [7]. The various health effects of some heavy metals will be highlighted below.

### 5.1 Arsenic

Arsenic exposure can lead to either acute or chronic toxicity. Acute arsenic poisoning can lead to the destruction of blood vessels, gastrointestinal tissue and can affect the heart and brain. Chronic arsenic toxicity which is termed arsenicosis usually focus on skin manifestations such as pigmentation and keratosis [81]. Lower level exposure to arsenic can cause nausea and vomiting, reduced production of erythrocytes and leukocytes and damage blood vessels, cause abnormal heart beat and pricking sensation in hands and legs. Long-term exposure can lead to the formation of skin lesions, pulmonary disease, neurological problems, peripheral vascular disease, diabetes mellitus, hypertension and cardiovascular disease [82]. Chronic arsenicosis may results to irreversible changes in the vital organs and possibly lead to death. Also, chronic arsenic exposure can promote the development of a number of cancers which include skin cancer, cancers of the bladder, lung, liver (angiosarcoma), and possibly the colon and kidney cancers [82]. Recently in the United States, the tolerable amount of arsenic in drinking water is 50 μg/liter but there is much concern of lowering this standard dose of population exposures to arsenic as the present dose is believed to increase the risk for cancer. Most environmental scientists studying this problem are of the view that the current tolerable limit of arsenic in drinking water or food be reduced.

### 5.2 Lead

Toxicity due to lead exposure is called lead poisoning. Lead poisoning is mostly related to the gastrointestinal tract and central nervous system in children and adults [83]. Lead poisoning can be either acute or chronic. Acute exposure of lead can cause headache, loss of appetite, abdominal pain, fatigue, sleeplessness, hallucinations, vertigo, renal dysfunction, hypertension and arthritis while chronic exposure can result in birth defects, mental retardation, autism, psychosis, allergies, paralysis, weight loss, dyslexia, hyperactivity, muscular weakness, kidney damage, brain damage, coma and may even cause death [81]. Although lead poisoning is preventable, it still remains a dangerous disease as it can affect most of the organs of the body. Exposure to elevated levels of lead can cause the plasma membrane of the blood brain barrier to move into the interstitial spaces leading to edema [84]. Also, lead exposure can disrupt the intracellular second messenger systems and alter the functioning of the central nervous system. Developing fetuses and children are most vulnerable to neurotoxic effects due to lead exposure. A number of prospective epidemiologic studies in children less than 5 years of age have shown that low-level of lead exposure (5–25 μg/dL in blood) resulted to the impairment of intellectual development which was manifested by the lost of intelligence quotient points [85]. As such, the Centers for Disease Control (CDC) in the United States has reduced the tolerable amount of lead in children's blood from 25 to 10 μg/dL and recommended universal screening of blood lead for all children.

### 5.3 Mercury

Mercury is an element that can easily combine with other elements to form inorganic and organic mercury. Exposure to elevated levels of metallic, inorganic and organic mercury can damage the kidney, brain and developing fetus [86] while methyl mercury is highly carcinogenic. Organic mercury is lipophilic in nature and thus can easily penetrate cell membranes. Mercury and its compound affects the nervous system and thus increased exposure of mercury can alter brain functions and lead to tremors, shyness, irritability, memory problems and changes in hearing or vision. Short-term exposure to metallic mercury vapors at higher levels can lead to vomiting, nausea, skin rashes, diarrhea, lung damage, high blood pressure, etc. while short-term exposure to organic mercury poisoning can lead to depression, tremors, headache, fatigue, memory problems, hair loss, etc. Since these symptoms are also common in other illness or disease conditions, diagnosis of mercury poisoning may be difficult in such cases [81]. Chronic levels of mercury exposure can lead to erethism, a disease condition characterized by excitability, tremor of the hands, memory loss, timidity, and insomnia. Also, occupational exposure to mercury as observed by researchers has been associated with measurable declines in performance on neurobehavioral tests of motor speed, visual scanning, visuomotor coordination, verbal and visual memory. Dimethylmercury is a very toxic compound that can penetrate the skin through latex gloves and its exposure at very low dose can cause the degeneration of the central nervous system and death. Mercury exposure to pregnant women can affect the fetus and offspring may suffer from mental retardation, cerebellar symptoms, retention of primitive reflexes, malformation and other abnormalities [87]. This has been confirmed in recent studies in which pregnant women exposed to mercury through dietary intake of whale meat and fish showed reduce motor neuron function, loss of memory, impaired speech and neural transmission in their offspring.

### 5.4 Cadmium

Cadmium and its compounds have several health effects in humans. The health effects of cadmium exposure are exacerbated due to the inability of the human body to excrete cadmium. In fact, cadmium is re-absorbed by the kidney thereby limiting its excretion. Short-term exposure to inhalation of cadmium can cause severe damages to the lungs and respiratory irritation while its ingestion in higher dose can cause stomach irritation resulting to vomiting and diarrhea. Long-term exposure to cadmium leads to its deposition in bones and lungs. As such, cadmium exposure can cause bone and lung damage [88]. Cadmium can cause bone mineralization as studies on animals and humans have revealed osteoporosis (skeletal damage) due to cadmium. It has been observed that “Itai-itai” disease, an epidemic of bone fractures in Japan is due to cadmium contamination [89]. Increased cadmium toxicity in this population was found to be associated with increased risk of bone fractures in women, as well as decreased bone density and height loss in males and females. Cadmium is highly toxic to the kidney and it accumulates in the proximal tubular cells in higher concentrations. Thus, cadmium exposure can cause renal dysfunction and kidney disease. Also, cadmium exposure can cause disturbances in calcium metabolism, formation of renal stones and hypercalciuria. Cadmium is also classified as group 1 carcinogens for humans by the International Agency for Research on Cancer. Tobacco is the main source of cadmium uptake in smokers and thus, smokers are more susceptible to cadmium intoxication than non-smokers [90]. Also, cadmium can cause testicular degeneration and a potential risk factor for prostate cancer.

### 5.5 Chromium

Chromium, in its hexavalent form, is the most toxic species of chromium though some other species such as Chromium (III) compounds are much less toxic and cause little or no health problems. Chromium (VI) has the tendency to be corrosive and also to cause allergic reactions to the body. Therefore, breathing high levels of chromium (VI) can cause irritation to the lining of the nose and nose ulcers. It can also cause anemia, irritations and ulcers in the small intestine and stomach, damage sperm and male reproductive system. The allergic reactions due to chromium include severe redness and swelling of the skin. Exposure of extremely high doses of chromium (VI) compounds to humans can result in severe cardiovascular, respiratory, hematological, gastrointestinal, renal, hepatic, and neurological effects and possibly death [91]. Exposure to chromium compounds can result in the formation of ulcers such as nasal septum ulcer which are very common in chromate workers. Exposure to higher amounts of chromium compounds in humans can lead to the inhibition of erythrocyte glutathione reductase, which in turn lowers the capacity to reduce methemoglobin to hemoglobin. *In vivo* and *in vitro* experiments have shown chromate compounds to induce DNA damage in many different ways and can lead to the formation of DNA adducts, chromosomal aberrations, alterations in replication sister chromatid exchanges, and transcription of DNA [92]. Thus, there are substantial evidence of chromium to promote carcinogenicity of humans as increase stomach tumors have been observed in animals and humans who were exposed to chromium(VI) in drinking water.

### 5.6 Iron

Iron salts such as iron sulfate, iron sulfate heptahydrate and iron sulfate monohydrate are of low acute toxicity when exposure is through dermal, oral and inhalation routes. However, other forms of iron are of serious health problems. Iron toxicity occurs in four stages. The first stage which commences 6 h after iron overdose is marked by gastrointestinal effects such as vomiting, diarrhea and gastro-intestinal bleeding. The progression to the second stage occurs 6–24 h after an overdose and it is considered as a latent period of apparent medical recovery. The third stage commences between 12 and 96 h after the onset of clinical symptoms and is characterized by hypotension, shocks, lethargy, hepatic necrosis, tachycardia, metabolic acidosis and may sometimes lead to death [93]. The fourth and final stage usually occurs within 2–6 weeks of iron overdose. This stage is marked by the development of strictures and formation of gastrointestinal ulcerations. Meat is rich in iron and thus meat eating countries are at risk of cancer as excess iron uptake increases the risk of cancer. Asbestos contains about 30% of iron and thus workers who are highly exposed to asbestos are at high risk of asbestosis, a condition which is known to cause lung cancer. Iron is known to generate free radicals which are suggested to be responsible for asbestos related cancer. Iron-induced free radicals can initiate cancer by the oxidation of DNA leading to DNA damage [94].

### 5.7 Manganese

Although manganese is an essential metal for the body, it recently became a metal of global concern when methylcyclopentadienyl manganese tricarbonyl (MMT), which was known to be toxic was introduced as a gasoline additive. MMT has been claimed to be an occupational manganese hazard and linked with the development of Parkinson's disease-like syndrome of tremour, gait disorder, postural instability, and cognitive disorder [95]. Exposure to elevated levels of manganese can result in neurotoxicity. Manganism is a neurological disease due to manganese characterized by rigidity, action tremour, a mask-like expression, gait disturbances, bradykinesia, micrographia, memory and cognitive dysfunction, and mood disorder [96]. The symptoms of manganism are very similar to that of Parkinson disease. However, the main differences between manganism and Parkinson disease is the insensitivity of manganism to levodopa (L-DOPA) administration and also the differences in the symptoms and progression of the disease [97].

## 6. Conclusion

The exposure of heavy metals to humans involve various diverse forms through food and water consumption, inhalation of polluted air, skin contact and most important by occupational exposure at workplace. Though some heavy metals such as iron and manganese are essential for certain biochemical and physiological activities in the body, elevated level in the body can have delirious health effects. Most of the other heavy metals are generally toxic to the body at very low level. The main mechanism of heavy metal toxicity include the generation of free radicals to cause oxidative stress, damage of biological molecules such as enzymes, proteins, lipids, and nucleic acids, damage of DNA which is key to carcinogenesis as well as neurotoxicity. Some of the heavy metal toxicity could be acute while others could be chronic after long-term exposure which may lead to the damage of several organs in the body such as the brain, lungs, liver, and kidney causing diseases in the body.

## Author details

Godwill Azeh Engwa[1*], Paschaline Udoka Ferdinand[2], Friday Nweke Nwalo[3] and Marian N. Unachukwu[4]

1 Biochemistry, Department of Chemical Sciences, Godfrey Okoye University, Enugu, Nigeria

2 Department of Environmental Biotechnology, Bio-resource Development Centre, National Biotechnology and Development Agency (NABDA), Abagana, Anambra State, Nigeria

3 Department of Biotechnology, Federal University, Ndufu-Alike Ikwo (FUNAI), Abakaliki, Nigeria

4 Department of Biological Sciences, Godfrey Okoye University, Enugu, Nigeria

*Address all correspondence to: engwagodwill@gmail.com

## References

[1] Duffus JH. Heavy metals—A meaningless term? Pure and Applied Chemistry. 2002;**74**(5):793-807

[2] Li F, Qiu ZZ, Zhang JD. Investigation, pollution mapping and simulative leakage health risk assessment for heavy metals and metalloids in groundwater from a typical brownfield, middle China. International Journal of Environmental Research and Public Health. 2017;**14**(7):768. DOI: 10.3390/ijerph14070768

[3] Bradl H, editor. Heavy Metals in the Environment: Origin, Interaction and Remediation. Vol. 6. London: Academic Press; 2002

[4] WHO/FAO/IAEA. Trace Elements in Human Nutrition and Health. Switzerland: Geneva: World Health Organization; 1996

[5] Florea A-M, Dopp E, Obe G, Rettenmeier AW. Genotoxicity of organometallic species. In: Hirner AV, Emons H, editors. Organic Metal and Metalloid Species in the Environment: Analysis, Distribution, Processes and Toxicological Evaluation. Heidelberg: Springer-Verlag; 2004. pp. 205-219

[6] Monisha J, Tenzin T, Naresh A, Blessy BM, Krishnamurthy NB. Toxicity, mechanism and health effects of some heavy metals. Interdisciplinary Toxicology. 2014;7(2):60-72

[7] Jarup L. Hazards of heavy metal contamination. British Medical Bulletin. 2003;**68**(1):167-182

[8] Krishna AK, Mohan KR. Distribution, correlation, ecological and health risk assessment of heavy metal contamination in surface soils around an industrial area, Hyderabad, India. Environment and Earth Science. 2016;**75**:411. DOI: 10.1007/s12665-015-5151-7

[9] Hu H. Human health and heavy metals exposure. In: McCally M, editor. Life Support: The Environment and Human Health. Massachusetts, USA: MIT Press; 2002

[10] Sauvé S. Time to revisit arsenic regulations: Comparing drinking water and rice. BMC Public Health. 2014;**14**:465

[11] Thurmer K, Williams E, Reutt-Robey J. Autocatalytic oxidation of lead crystallite surfaces. Science. 2002;**297**(5589):2033-2035

[12] Wani AL, Ara A, Usmani JA. Lead toxicity: A review. Interdisciplinary Toxicology. 2015;**8**(2):55-64

[13] Rahimzadeh MR, Rahimzadeh MR, Kazemi S, Moghadamnia A. Cadmium toxicity and treatment: An update. Caspian Journal of Internal Medicine. 2017;**8**(3):135-145

[14] Unaegbu M, Engwa GA, Abaa QD, Aliozo SO, Ayuk EL, Osuji GA, et al. Heavy metal, nutrient and antioxidant status of selected fruit samples sold in Enugu, Nigeria. International Journal of Food Contamination. 2016;**3**(7):1-8

[15] Engwa AG, Ihekwoaba CJ, Ilo US, Unaegbu M, Ayuk LE, Osuji AG. Determination of some soft drink constituents and contamination by some heavy metals in Nigeria. Toxicology Reports. 2015;**2**:384-390

[16] Ghani A. Effect of chromium toxicity on growth, chlorophyll and some mineral nutrients of *Brassica juncea* L. Egyptian Acadmic Journal of Biological Sciences. 2011;**2**(1):9-15

[17] Zayed AM, Terry N. Chromium in the environment: Factors affecting biological remediation. Plant and Soil. 2003;**249**(1):139-156

[18] Agency for Toxic Substances and Disease Registry (ATSDR). Toxicological Profile for Copper. Atlanta: U.S. Department of Health and Humans Services, Public Health Service, Centers for Diseases Control; 2004

[19] Ferner DJ. Toxicity, heavy metals. eMedical Journal. 2001;**2**(5):1-8

[20] Ming-Ho Y. Environmental Toxicology: Biological and Health Effects of Pollutants, Chap.12. 2nd ed. Boca Raton, USA: CRC Press LLC; 2005 ISBN 1-56670-670-2

[21] Florea A-M, Busselberg D. Occurrence, use and potential toxic effects of metals and metal compounds. Biometals. 2006;**19**:419-427

[22] Valko M, Morris H, MTD C. Metals, toxicity and oxidative stress. Current Medicinal Chemistry. 2005;**12**:1161-1208

[23] Valko M, Izakovic M, Mazur M, Rhodes CJ, Telser J. Role of oxygen radicals in DNA damage and cancer incidence. Molecular and Cellular Biochemistry. 2004;**266**:37-56

[24] Bucher JR, Tien M, Aust SD. The requirement for ferric in the initiation of lipid peroxidation by chelated ferrous iron. Biochemistry and Biophysical Research Communication. 1983;**111**:777-784

[25] Eaton JW, Qian MW. Molecular bases of cellular iron toxicity. Free Radical Biology Medicine. 2002;**32**:833-840

[26] Lloyd RV, Hanna PM, Mason RP. The origin of the hydroxyl radical oxygen in the Fenton reaction. Free Radical Biology and Medicine. 1997;**22**:885-888

[27] Brezova V, Valko M, Breza M, Morris H, Telser J, Dvoranova D, et al. Role of radicals and singlet oxygen in photoactivated DNA cleavage by the anticancer drug camptothecin: An electron paramagnetic resonance study. Physical Chemistry B. 2003;**107**:2415-2425

[28] Burkitt MJ. A critical overview of the chemistry of copper-dependent low density lipoprotein oxidation: Roles of lipid hydroperoxides, α-tocopherol, thiols, and ceruloplasmin. Archive of Biochemistry and Biophysics. 2001;**394**:117-135

[29] Liu KJ, Shi XL. In vivo reduction of chromium (VI) and its related free radical generation. Molecular and Cellular Biochemistry. 2001;**222**:41-47

[30] Hanna PM, Kadiiska MB, Mason RP. Oxygen-derived free-radical and active oxygen complex-formation from cobalt (II) chelates in vitro. Chemistry Research Toxicology. 1992;**5**:109-115

[31] Crans DC, Smee JJ, Gaidamauskas E, Yang LQ. The chemistry and biochemistry of vanadium and the biological activities exerted by vanadium compounds. Chemistry Review. 2004;**104**:849-902

[32] Pi J, Horiguchi S, Sun Y, Nikaido M, Shimojo N, Hayashi T, et al. A potential mechanism for the impairment of nitric oxide formation caused by prolonged oral exposure to arsenate in rabbits. Free Radical Biology and Medicine. 2003;**35**:102-113

[33] Rin K, Kawaguchi K, Yamanaka K, Tezuka M, Oku N, Okada S. DNA-strand breaks induced by dimethylarsinic acid, a metabolite of inorganic arsenics, are strongly enhanced by superoxide anion radicals. Biology and Pharmacology Bulletin. 1995;**18**:45-48

[34] Kim HS, Kim YJ, Seo YR. An overview of carcinogenic heavy metal: Molecular toxicity mechanism and prevention. Journal of Cancer Prevention. 2015;**20**:232-240

[35] Chen J. The cell-cycle arrest and apoptotic functions of p53 in tumor initiation and progression. Cold Spring Harbor Perspectives in Medicine. 2016;**6**(1-6):a026104

[36] Martinez VD, Vucic EA, Becker-Santos DD, Gil L, Lam WL. Arsenic exposure and the induction of human cancers. Journal of Toxicology. 2011;**2011**:1-13

[37] Bjørklund G, Aaseth J, Chirumbolo S, Urbina MA, Uddin R. Efects of arsenic toxicity beyond epigenetic modiications. Environmental Geochemistry and Health. 2017;**39**:1-11

[38] Park YH, Kim D, Dai J, Zhang Z. Human bronchial epithelial BEAS-2B cells, an appropriate in vitro model to study heavy metals induced carcinogenesis. Toxicology and Applied Pharmacology. 2015;**287**(3):240-245

[39] Saleha Banu B, Danadevi K, Jamil K, Ahuja YR, Visweswara Rao K, Ishaq M. In vivo genotoxic effect of arsenic trioxide in mice using comet assay. Toxicology. 2001;**162**:171-177

[40] Hartwig A, Schwerdtle T. Interactions by carcinogenic metal compounds with DNA repair processes: Toxicological implications. Toxicology Letter. 2002;**127**:47-54

[41] García-Esquinas E, Pollán M, Umans JG, Francesconi KA, Goessler W, Guallar E. Arsenic exposure and cancer mortality in a US-based prospective cohort: The strong heart study. Cancer Epidemiology, Biomarkers & Prevention. 2013;**22**:1944-1953

[42] Silbergeld EK, Waalkes M, Rice JM. Lead as a carcinogen: Experimental evidence and mechanisms of action. American Journal of Industrial Medicine. 2000;**38**(3):316-323

[43] Crespo-Lopez ME, Macedo GL, Pereira SI, Arrifano GP, Picanco-Diniz DL, do Nascimento JL, et al. Mercury and human genotoxicity: Critical considerations and possible molecular mechanisms. Pharmacological Research. 2009;**60**(4):212-220

[44] Zhou C, Huang C, Wang J, Huang H, Li J, Xie Q, et al. LncRNA MEG3 downregulation mediated by DNMT3b contributes to nickel malignant transformation of human bronchial epithelial cells via modulating PHLPP1 transcription and HIF-1α translation. Oncogene. 2017;**36**:3878-3889

[45] Zambelli B, Uversky VN, Ciurli S. Nickel impact on human health: An intrinsic disorder perspective. Biochimica Et Biophysica Acta (BBA) – Proteins and Proteomics. 2016;**1864**(12):1714-1731

[46] Neal AP, Guilarte TR. Mechanisms of heavy metal neurotoxicity: Lead and manganese. Journal of Drug Metabolism and Toxicology. 2012;**S5**:002

[47] Nihei MK, Desmond NL, McGlothan JL, Kuhlmann AC, Guilarte TR. N-methyl-D-aspartate receptor subunit changes are associated with lead induced deficits of long-term potentiation and spatial learning. Neuroscience. 2000;**99**:233-242

[48] Morris RG, Garrud P, Rawlins JN, O'Keefe J. Place navigation impaired in rats with hippocampal lesions. Nature. 1982;**297**:681-683

[49] Tsien JZ, Huerta PT, Tonegawa S. The essential role of hippocampal CA1 NMDA receptor-dependent synaptic plasticity in spatial memory. Cell. 1996;**87**:1327-1338

[50] Alkondon M, Costa AC, Radhakrishnan V, Aronstam RS, Albuquerque EX. Selective blockade of NMDA-activated channel currents may be implicated in learning deficits caused by lead. FEBS Letters. 1990;**261**:124-130

[51] Neal AP, Worley PF, Guilarte TR. Lead exposure during synaptogenesis alters NMDA receptor targeting via NMDA receptor inhibition. Neurotoxicology. 2011;**32**:281-289

[52] Guilarte TR, Miceli RC, Jett DA. Neurochemical aspects of hippocampal and cortical $Pb^{2+}$ neurotoxicity. Neurotoxicology. 1994;**15**:459-466

[53] Neal AP, Guilarte TR. Molecular neurobiology of lead (Pb(2+)): Effects on synaptic function. Molecular Neurobiology. 2010;**42**:151-160

[54] Fayyazuddin A, Villarroel A, Le Goff A, Lerma J, Neyton J. Four residues of the extracellular N-terminal domain of the NR2A subunit control high-affinity $Zn^{2+}$ binding to NMDA receptors. Neuron. 2000;**25**:685-694

[55] Xu SZ, Rajanna B. Glutamic acid reverses Pb2+–induced reductions of NMDA receptor subunits in vitro. Neurotoxicology. 2006;**27**:169-175

[56] Guilarte TR, McGlothan JL, Nihei MK. Hippocampal expression of N-methyl-D-aspartate receptor (NMDAR1) subunit splice variant mRNA is altered by developmental exposure to Pb2+. Molecular Brain Research. 2000;**76**:299-305

[57] Guilarte TR, McGlothan JL. Selective decrease in NR1 subunit splice variant mRNA in the hippocampus of $Pb^{2+-}$exposed rats: Implications for synaptic targeting and cell surface expression of NMDAR complexes. Brain Research and Molecular Brain Research. 2003;**113**:37-43

[58] Lasley SM, Gilbert ME. Presynaptic glutamatergic function in dentate gyrus in vivo is diminished by chronic exposure to inorganic lead. Brain Research. 1996;**736**:125-134

[59] Xiao C, Gu Y, Zhou CY, Wang L, Zhang MM. Pb2+ impairs GABAergic synaptic transmission in rat hippocampal slices: A possible involvement of presynaptic calcium channels. Brain Research. 2006;**1088**:93-100

[60] Braga MF, Pereira EF, Albuquerque EX. Nanomolar concentrations of lead inhibit glutamatergic and GABAergic transmission in hippocampal neurons. Brain Research. 1999;**826**:22-34

[61] Peng S, Hajela RK, Atchison WD. Characteristics of block by $Pb^{2+}$ of function of human neuronal L-, N-, and R-type $Ca^{2+}$ channels transiently expressed in human embryonic kidney 293 cells. Molecular Pharmacology. 2002;**62**:1418-1430

[62] Waites CL, Garner CC. Presynaptic function in health and disease. Trends in Neuroscience. 2011;**34**:326-337

[63] Mirnics K, Middleton FA, Lewis DA, Levitt P. Analysis of complex brain disorders with gene expression microarrays: Schizophrenia as a disease of the synapse. Trends in Neuroscience. 2001;**24**:479-486

[64] Konur S, Ghosh A. Calcium signaling and the control of dendritic development. Neuron. 2005;**46**:401-405

[65] Milatovic D, Gupta RC, Yin Z, Zaja-Milatovic S, Aschner M. Manganese in Reproductive and Developmental Toxicology. 2017. pp. 567-581. DOI: 10.1016/B978-0-12-804239-7.00032-9

[66] Chen JY, Tsao GC, Zhao Q, Zheng W. Differential cytotoxicity of Mn(II) and Mn(III): Special reference to mitochondrial [Fe-S] containing enzymes. Toxicology and Applied Pharmacology. 2001;**175**:160-168

[67] Gunter TE, Gerstner B, Lester T, Wojtovich AP, Malecki J. An analysis of the effects of $Mn^{2+}$ on oxidative

phosphorylation in liver, brain, and heart mitochondria using state 3 oxidation rate assays. Toxicology Applied Pharmacology. 2010;**249**:65-75

[68] Milatovic D, Zaja-Milatovic S, Gupta RC, Yu Y, Aschner M. Oxidative damage and neurodegeneration in manganese-induced neurotoxicity. Toxicology and Applied Pharmacology. 2009;**240**:219-225

[69] Gunter TE, Gavin CE, Aschner M, Gunter KK. Speciation of manganese in cells and mitochondria: A search for the proximal cause of manganese neurotoxicity. Neurotoxicology. 2006;**27**:765-776

[70] Paris I, Segura-Aguilar J. The role of metal ions in dopaminergic neuron degernation in parkinsonism and Parkinson's disease. Monatsh Chemistry. 2011;**142**:365-374

[71] Burton NC, Guilarte TR. Manganese neurotoxicity: Lessons learned from longitudinal studies in nonhuman primates. Environmental Health Perspectives. 2009;**117**:325-332211

[72] Benedetto A, Au C, Avila DS, Milatovic D, Aschner M. Extracellular dopamine potentiates mn-induced oxidative stress, lifespan reduction, and dopaminergic neurodegeneration in a BLI-3-dependent manner in *Caenorhabditis elegans*. PLoS Genetics. 2010;**6**:e1001084

[73] Chrestensen CA, Starke DW, Mieyal JJ. Acute cadmium exposure inactivates thioltransferase (Glutaredoxin), inhibits intracellular reduction of protein-glutathionyl-mixed disulfides, and initiates apoptosis. The Journal of Biological Chemistry. 2000;**275**:26556-26565

[74] Duruibe JO, Ogwuegbu MO, Egwurugwu JN. Heavy metal pollution and human biotoxic effects. International Journal of Physical Sciences. 2007;**2**(5):112-118

[75] Naganuma A, Miura N, Kaneko S, Mishina T, Hosoya S, Miyairi S, et al. GFAT as a target molecule of methylmercury toxicity in *Saccharomyces cerevisiae*. FASEB Journal. 2000;**14**:968-972

[76] Hartwig A. Zinc finger proteins as potential targets for toxic metal ions: Differential effects on structure and function. Antioxidant Redox Signal. 2001;**3**:625-634

[77] Faller P, Kienzler K, Krieger-Liszkay A. Mechanism of $Cd^{2+}$ toxicity: $Cd^{2+}$ inhibits photoactivation of photosystem II by competitive binding to the essential $Ca^{2+}$ site. Biochemical Biophysics Acta. 2005;**1706**:158-164

[78] Sharma SK, Goloubinoff P, Christen P. Heavy metal ions are potent inhibitors of protein folding. Biochemical and Biophysics Research Communication. 2008;**372**:341-345

[79] Tamás MJ, Sharma SK, Ibstedt S, Jacobson T, Christen P. Heavy metals and metalloids As a cause for protein misfolding and aggregation. Biomolecules. 2014;**4**:252-267

[80] Jacobson T, Navarrete C, Sharma SK, Sideri TC, Ibstedt S, Priya S, et al. Arsenite interferes with protein folding and triggers formation of protein aggregates in yeast. Journal of Cell Science. 2012;**125**:5073-5083

[81] Martin S, Griswold W. Human health effects of heavy metals. Environmental Science and Technology Briefs for Citizens. 2009;**15**:1-6

[82] Huy TB, Tuyet-Hanh TT, Johnston R, Nguyen-Viet H. Assessing health risk due to exposure to arsenic in drinking water in Hanam Province, Vietnam. International Journal of Environmental Research and Public Health. 2014;**11**:7575-7591

[83] Markowitz M. Lead poisoning. Pediatry Review. 2000;**21**(10):327-335

[84] Teo J, Goh K, Ahuja A, Ng H, Poon W. Intracranial vascular calcifi cations, glioblastoma multiforme, and lead poisoning. American Journal of Neuroradiology. 1997;**18**:576-579

[85] Brown MJ, Margolis S. Lead in drinking water and human blood Lead levels in the United States. In: The Morbidity and Mortality Weekly Report (MMWR). Washington, DC: Center for Disease Control and Prevention (CDC); 2012

[86] Alina M, Azrina A, Mohd Yunus AS, Mohd Zakiuddin S, Mohd Izuan Effendi H, Muhammad Rizal R. Heavy metals (mercury, arsenic, cadmium, plumbum) in selected marine fi sh and shellfi sh along the straits of Malacca. International Food Research Journal. 2012;**19**(1):135-140

[87] Bernhoft RA. Mercury toxicity and treatment: A review of the literature. International Journal of Environmental Research and Public Health. 2012;**2012**:1-10

[88] Bernard A. Cadmium & its adverse effects on human health. Indian Journal Medical Research. 2008;**128**(4):557-564

[89] Nishijo M, Nakagawa H, Suwazono Y, Nogawa K, Kido T. Causes of death in patients with Itaiitai disease suffering from severe chronic cadmium poisoning: A nested case-control analysis of a follow-up study in Japan. BMJ Open. 2017;7:e015694

[90] Mudgal V, Madaan N, Mudgal A, Singh RB, Mishra S. Effect of toxic metals on human health. Open Nutraceuticals Journal. 2010;**3**:94-99

[91] Shekhawat K, Chatterjee S, Joshi B. Chromium toxicity and its health hazards. International Journal of Advanced Research. 2015;7(3):167-172

[92] Matsumoto ST, Mantovani MS, Malaguttii MIA, Dias AL, Fonseca IC, Marin-Morales MA. Genotoxicity and mutagenicity of water contaminated with tannery effluents, as evaluated by the micronucleus test and comet assay using the fish *Oreochromis niloticus* and chromosome aberrations in onion root-tips. Genetics Molecular Biology. 2006;**29**(1):148-158

[93] Hillman RS. Hematopoietic agents: Growth factors, minerals, and vitamins. In: Hardman JG, Limbird LE, Gilman AG, editors. Goodman & Gilman's the Pharmacological Basis of Therapeutics. 10th ed. New York: McGraw-Hill; 2001. pp. 1487-1518

[94] Bhasin G, Kauser H, Athar M. Iron augments stage-I and stage-II tumor promotion in murine skin. Cancer Letter. 2002;**183**(2):113-122

[95] O'Neal S, Zheng W. Manganese toxicity upon overexposure: A decade in review. USA. Current Environmental Health Reports. 2015;**2**:315-328

[96] Klos KJ, Chandler M, Kumar N, Ahlskog JE, Josephs KA. Neuropsychological profiles of manganese neurotoxicity. European Journal of Neurology. 2006;**13**:1139-1141

[97] Guilarte TR. Manganese and Parkinson's disease: A critical review and new findings. Environmental Health Perspectives. 2010;**118**:1071-1080

Chapter 6

# Nephrotoxic Effects of Drugs

*Azade Sari*


## Abstract

Drug-induced nephrotoxicity is a renal dysfunction that occurs as a result of exposure to nephrotoxic drugs. It is a common problem in certain clinical situations such as underlying renal dysfunction, cardiovascular disease, diabetes, and sepsis. Drugs can cause mild to moderate nephrotoxic problems such as intrarenal obstruction, interstitial nephritis, nephrotic syndrome, acid-base and fluid-electrolyte disturbances, alteration in intraglomerular hemodynamics, inflammatory changes in renal tubular cells, tubulointerstitial disease, and renal scarring leading to acute or chronic kidney injury. Therefore, early detection of adverse effects of drugs as well as the clinical history of the patient, basic renal functions, drug-related risk factors, and nephrotoxic drug combinations must be well known in order to prevent drug-induced nephrotoxicity and progression to end-stage renal disease.


**Keywords:** nephrotoxicity, drugs, drug interaction, acute kidney injury, chronic kidney injury, prevention strategies, nephrotoxicity biomarkers

## 1. Introduction

Acute kidney injury is the deterioration of the renal function over hours or days, resulting in the accumulation of toxic wastes and the loss of internal homeostasis. It can be caused by numerous etiologies [1, 2], and medications are a relatively common cause of kidney injury among these injuries [3]. Drug-induced nephrotoxicity is a renal dysfunction that occurs as a result of direct or indirect exposure to nephrotoxic prescribed drugs, over-the-counter products, diagnostic agents, or alternative/complementary products (herbal remedies, natural products, nutritional supplements) that are widely available at most health food stores [3, 4]. Drug-induced nephrotoxicity is an extremely common condition and is responsible for a variety of pathological effects on the kidneys [4]. Nephrotoxicity most commonly affects tubulointerstitial compartment and manifests either acute tubular injury (ATI) or acute interstitial nephritis (AIN). There is a growing incidence of drug-induced glomerular disease, including direct cellular injury and immune-mediated injury [5]. However, kidney disease does not develop in all patients exposed to the various potential nephrotoxins [3]. The nephrotoxicity of medications, drugs, or other ingested substances is a complicated process that involves a combination of factors.

Potential nephrotoxic effect of the drug, comorbid diseases or conditions (underlying renal dysfunction, cardiovascular disease, diabetes, immunologic diseases, sepsis, etc.), genetic determinants of drug metabolism and transport, immune response genes, drug dose and duration of therapy, drug characteristics (solubility, structure and charge), combinations of potential nephrotoxic drugs, urine pH, metabolic disturbances, older age (>65 year), and female sex are the common risk factors for drug-induced nephrotoxicity [1–5].

## 2. Preventive measures of drug-induced nephropathy

Basic renal functions should be evaluated and patient's renal functions should be considered when prescribing a new drug.

Dosage adjustments of the drugs should be done according to the patient's basic renal functions.

Risk factors for nephrotoxicity must be corrected before initiation of therapy.

Nephrotoxic drug combination should be avoided.

Adequate hydration before and during therapy must be ensured.

Whenever possible, equally effective nonnephrotoxic drugs should be used [4].

## 3. Biomarkers of drug-induced kidney injury

Early detection of drug-induced kidney injury is vital. Traditional biomarkers such as creatinine (Cr) and blood urea nitrogen (BUN) are insensitive for monitoring renal safety. Thus, new biomarkers have been investigated for accurate diagnosis, risk assessment, adopting therapy, and improvement of clinical outcome. [4, 6–9] Serum Cr can raise in prerenal azotemia without tubular injury, and some factors such as muscle mass, total body weight, fluid status, age, gender, race, and drugs influence serum Cr levels [8]. There are novel biomarkers that are more sensitive and can detect renal damage earlier than serum BUN and Cr levels [4, 6–9]. It is clear that which marker indicates kidney damage, but it is not yet clear when they should be measured. Also it is not clear if these biomarkers should be used for clinical decision-making or what should be done when the levels are elevated. Further studies are required for the routine clinical use of these biomarkers [8]. **Table 1** lists common novel biomarkers that are under investigation.

### 3.1 Neutrophil gelatinase-associated lipocalin (NGAL)

NGAL is an acute phase reactant, and it can raise in inflammatory conditions. It is expressed by tubular epithelial cells in response to injury and tubulointerstitial damage. It can be measured in both plasma and urine [8–13], but for early detection of acute kidney injury (AKI), increase in urine NGAL is more specific than increase in plasma NGAL [9]. Baseline renal functions, severity of AKI, and age influence the level of NGAL. Studies showed that plasma and urine NGAL levels rise 2 hours after the injury; thus, it is the strongest predictor of AKI [8, 9]. It is more sensitive in ischemic and toxic (tacrolimus, cisplatin, cyclosporine A, radiographic contrast agent) AKI. [9] NGAL levels can be a predictor of clinical outcomes of AKI (need for dialysis and mortality) [9, 11] and progression of chronic kidney disease (CKD) in adults [8, 10, 12, 13]. Urine excretion of NGAL may be increased by albuminuria [9].

### 3.2 Cystatin-C (Cys-C)

Cys-C is a protein that synthesized in all nucleated cells. It is freely filtered in the glomerulus and reabsorbed and catabolized completely in the proximal tubules without tubular secretion. It is an alternative parameter of serum Cr in the measurement of renal function [8–11, 13]. Serum Cys-C levels are not influenced

| Biomarker | Source | Region specificity | Clinical application |
|---|---|---|---|
| NGAL | Plasma/urine | Proximal tubule/distal tubule | AKI/CKD |
| Cyclophilins | Urine | Glomerulus/proximal tubule | AKI |
| KIM-1 | Urine | Proximal tubule | AKI/CKD |
| IL-18 | Urine | Proximal tubule | AKI |
| L-FABP | Urine | Proximal tubule | AKI |
| H-FABP | Plasma/urine | Distal tubule | AKI |
| NAG | Urine | Proximal tubule | AKI |
| α-GST | Urine | Proximal tubule | AKI |
| π-GST | Urine | Distal tubule | AKI |
| γ-GT | Urine | Proximal tubule | AKI |
| Low-molecular-weight proteins | | | |
| *Cystatin-C* | Urine | Glomerulus/proximal tubule | AKI |
| *$\alpha_1$-Microglobulin* | Urine | Proximal tubule/glomerulus | AKI/CKD |
| *$\beta_2$-Microglobulin* | Urine | Proximal tubule | AKI/CKD |
| *RBP* | Urine | Proximal tubule | AKI |
| Cell cycle arrest proteins | | | |
| *IGFBP-7* | Urine | Proximal tubule | AKI |
| *TIMP-2* | Urine | Proximal tubule | AKI |
| Clusterin | Urine | Proximal tubule/distal tubule | AKI/CKD |
| TFF-3 | Urine | Proximal tubule/distal tubule | AKI/CKD |

**Table 1.**
*Summary of novel nephrotoxicity biomarkers.*

by gender, age, total body weight, muscle mass, or race, but tubular reabsorption is decreased by marked albuminuria [9–11]. It is thought to be the best biomarker for early kidney injury and more reliable marker of renal function [8, 10, 11].

### 3.3 Cyclophilins

They are structural proteins and measured in urine and plasma. Elevated levels of cyclophilins indicate AKI [11].

### 3.4 Kidney injury molecule-1 (KIM-1)

KIM-1 is a transmembrane glycoprotein. After ischemic or toxic injury, its levels elevate and it helps to distinguish acute tubular nephritis (ATN) from prerenal azotemia and CKD. Elevated urine KIM-1 levels are highly specific for kidney injury, because it is only expressed in injured kidney [8–13]. Some studies suggest KIM-1 as an indicator of AKI transition to CKD, because high levels of KIM-1 are maintained during CKD progression [12].

### 3.5 Interleukin-18 (IL-18)

It is also known as interferon-γ (IFN-γ)-inducing factor and its urinary levels rise in ischemic and toxic AKI [9]. It predicts renal parenchymal injury [10]. Its levels are higher in patients with ATN. Increased urinary levels of IL-18 are a predictor of poor outcome such as death and the need for short-term dialysis [8, 9]. According to some studies, urine IL-18 levels increase in contrast-induced AKI [12], 6–12 hours after administration of the radiocontrast agent [9].

### 3.6 Cell cycle arrest biomarkers

Insulin-like growth factor-binding protein 7 (IGFBP-7) and tissue inhibitor of metalloproteinase-2 (TIMP-2) are the two biomarkers included in this group. They are measured in urine and can be used for risk stratification of AKI [8, 9]. According to some studies, the most important advantage of these biomarkers is that their levels are not affected by comorbid diseases such as CKD, diabetes, and sepsis [8].

### 3.7 Liver-type fatty acid-binding protein (L-FABP)

FABP is a cytoplasmic protein found in all tissues with fatty acid metabolism. In kidneys, liver-type (in proximal tubule) and heart-type (in distal tubule) FABP present. Studies showed that urinary L-FABP is a useful biomarker in ischemic and toxic (especially cisplatin toxicity and contrast-induced nephropathy) AKI [9, 10, 12]. Elevated urinary and plasma H-FABP levels are indicator of distal tubular injury [10].

### 3.8 N-acetyl-beta-D glucosaminidase (NAG)

It is an enzyme produced by the proximal tubular cells. It can be found in the urine in very small amounts in healthy people. It cannot be filtered by glomerulus; thus, elevated levels of urine NAG indicate tubular damage [9, 10, 12]. Studies showed that NAG is a useful, sensitive, and early biomarker of contrast-induced AKI and high urinary levels correlate with poor outcome [9]. Also, high urinary NAG levels have been showed to be an indicator of clinical and subclinical tubular damage after chemotherapy [10] and are a sensitive biomarker of acute oxidative stress [11].

### 3.9 Midkine

It is a heparin-binding growth factor. Although not studied well, it may increase in contrast-induced AKI [9].

### 3.10 α- and π-glutathione S-transferase (α-GST, π-GST)

They are cytosolic, microsomal, and membrane-bound enzymes. They are detoxification enzymes that present in kidney and many other organs. Some studies showed elevation in urine α-GST indicating epithelial necrosis in the proximal tubules and π-GST indicating epithelial necrosis in the distal tubules [9–11]. α-GST is thought to be a biomarker of proximal tubular necrosis of cisplatin-induced injury. α-GST and KIM-1 are sensitive biomarkers for predicting polymyxin-induced nephrotoxicity [10].

### 3.11 γ-Glutamil transpeptidase (γGT) and alkaline phosphatase (AP)

They are two enzymes that may increase in urine in proximal tubular epithelial damage [9–11]. Some studies showed increased levels of γGT, 24 hours after contrast administration [9], and some showed that it may be a sensitive biomarker of acute paracetamol nephrotoxicity [11].

Alanine amino peptidase (AAP), lactate dehydrogenase (LDH), β-galactosidase, β-glucuronidase, and leucine aminopeptidase are the other enzymes that are used for nephrotoxicity biomarkers [10, 11].

### 3.12 β-2-Microglobulin

It is a low-molecular-weight protein. It is normally found in urine but increases in tubular injury secondary to antibiotic, analgesic, solvent, heavy metal, or pesticide poisoning. In these conditions, it has been proved to be a sensitive biomarker of renal tubular damage [9–13]. But it rapidly degrades in room temperature and urine $pH < 6$; therefore, its utility as a urinary biomarker is limited [12].

### 3.13 α-1-Microglobulin

It is a low-molecular-weight protein, and elevated urinary levels can be used as a biomarker of tubular injury [10–12]. It is resistant to pH changes; thus, it is a sensitive biomarker of proximal tubular dysfunction [12].

### 3.14 Retinol-binding protein (RBP)

It is a low-molecular-weight protein that functions in vitamin A transportation from the liver to other tissues. It is a sensitive biomarker in proximal tubular damage [9–11].

### 3.15 MicroRNA (miRNA)

Although not demonstrated well, some subgroups of miRNA (miRNA-30a, -30c, and -30e) may rise in serum and urine in the states of contrast-induced AKI [9].

### 3.16 Clusterin

It is a glycoprotein and may be used as a biomarker for cisplatin-induced nephrotoxicity [10]. Urinary clusterin levels may increase following drug-induced nephrotoxicity [13].

### 3.17 Trefoil factor 3 (TFF3)

It is another new biomarker of nephrotoxicity that is mainly expressed in kidneys. Studies showed marked decrease in urinary TFF3 after nephrotoxic AKI [13].

## 4. Common nephrotoxic drugs

### 4.1 Antibiotics

#### *4.1.1 β-Lactam antibiotics*

β-Lactam antibiotics include penicillins, cephalosporins, cephamycins, carbapenems, monobactams, and β-lactamase inhibitors, and these are among the most commonly prescribed antibiotics [14]. β-Lactam antibiotics, especially penicillins and cephalosporins, frequently cause hypersensitivity reactions. Methicillin and nafcillin are the prototypical drugs for hypersensitivity reactions associated with AIN. It is generally characterized by acute and severe renal failure. Hematuria, proteinuria, leucocyturia, and pyuria are seen in urinary sediment of affected patients. Hypersensitivity reactions such as fever, rush, and peripheral eosinophilia are commonly seen [5, 14].

Piperacillin-tazobactam and vancomycin must not be used concurrently; they may cause AKI. Cephalosporins may exacerbate the renal toxicity of aminoglycosides [14].

#### *4.1.2 Non-β-lactam antibiotics*

They can cause AIN. Rifampicin-induced AIN is dose dependent and is commonly associated with oliguric acute renal failure, hemolytic anemia, thrombocytopenia, and hepatitis. Approximately two-thirds of patients affected by rifampin-induced AIN require renal transplantation [5].

#### *4.1.3 Aminoglycosides*

Aminoglycosides are antibiotics used in the treatment of Gram-negative and *Staphylococcus aureus* infections [1]. Aminoglycosides commonly cause acute kidney injury during therapy. It typically manifests after 5–7 days of therapy. It is described as a rise in the plasma creatinine concentration of more than 0.5–1 mg/dL or 50% increase in plasma creatinine concentration from baseline [15].

Tubular uptake of aminoglycosides is a saturable process; thus, a single daily high dose is preferable to divided low doses. Administration of aminoglycosides by this way will cause less nephrotoxic effect [4, 15, 16].

Aminoglycosides primarily affect proximal tubules [1, 16], and patients present with acute tubular necrosis, showing features such as nonoliguric acute renal failure [4]. Proximal dysfunction leads to loss of enzymes, proteins, glucose, calcium, potassium, and magnesium [1]. In some patients, distal tubular segments can be affected and this manifests as polyuria and hypomagnesemia. Most patients may recover but some progress to irreversible kidney damage, especially if the patient is hypovolemic, septic, or catabolic. Aminoglycoside nephrotoxicity risk factors are nearly the same as other nephrotoxic agents. In addition to common factors, higher creatinine clearances and hypoalbuminemia are also independent risk factors for aminoglycoside nephrotoxicity [9].

#### *4.1.4 Polymyxins/colistin*

Polymyxins are a group of antibiotics that are used for pan-resistant nosocomial infections, especially for *Pseudomonas* and *Acinetobacter* spp. They may cause nephrotoxicity by IV injection. The nephrotoxicity mechanism is ATN leading to acute renal failure (ARF) with hematuria, proteinuria, and oliguria.

According to data, colistin appears more nephrotoxic than polymyxin B. Colistin-induced nephrotoxicity may exacerbate by older age, preexisting renal insufficiency, hypoalbuminemia, and concomitant use of NSAIDs. There are limited data on the risk factors for polymyxin-B associated nephrotoxicity. Methoxyflurane and cefazedone may enhance the nephrotoxic effect of polymyxin-B. Methoxyflurane-polymyxin-B combination should be avoided, but polymyxin-B-cefazedone combination may be used by close monitoring renal functions. Also, polymyxin-B may enhance the nephrotoxic effect of bacitracin [17, 18].

### 4.2 Analgesics

Analgesic nephropathy is a CKD characterized by papillary necrosis and chronic interstitial nephritis. It is caused by prolonged consumption of analgesic agents. Hypertension is a common clinical finding. The major laboratory manifestations are hematuria, sterile pyuria, elevation in serum Cr levels, and anemia [19, 20].

#### *4.2.1 Nonsteroidal anti-inflammatory drugs (NSAIDs)*

NSAIDs lead to AIN, chronic interstitial nephritis and finally CKD [20, 21]. Risk factors that may increase the nephrotoxic effect of NSAIDs are congestive heart failure, age > 65 years, and preexisting renal disease [4, 21].

#### *4.2.2 Acetylsalicylic acid (ASA)*

When used alone, even if prolonged, acetylsalicylic acid is not thought to cause kidney damage. It aggravates the nephrotoxic effects of both phenacetin and acetaminophen; thus, it should not be used simultaneously with these drugs. Acetylsalicylic acid and acetaminophen combination leads to papillary necrosis and calcification. Acetylsalicylic acid and NSAID combination leads to ischemic injury [20].

#### *4.2.3 Acetaminophen (paracetamol)*

Oral and rectal forms of acetaminophen may cause nephrotoxicity with chronic overdose [12]. The incidence of renal dysfunction is related to the severity of the acetaminophen ingestion [22]. IV forms may cause oliguria in neonates, infants, children, and adults [23]. AKI, which is primarily ATN, is manifested by elevations of BUN and Cr along with proteinuria, hematuria, and granular and epithelial cell casts on urine analyses. Also vascular endothelial damage can occur. It may be used in severe renal impairment with caution and dosing must be adjusted. Renal functions spontaneously return to baseline within 1–4 weeks. Rarely dialysis may be required. There is no evidence that N-acetylcysteine has any protective effect on nephrotoxicity [22, 23].

### 4.3 5-Aminosalicylates (5-ASAs)

5-ASAs are used to treat inflammatory bowel diseases. They lead hypersensitivity reactions in multiple organs, especially in kidneys, leading to acute interstitial nephritis [5, 24, 25]. During 5-ASA therapy, regular monitoring of renal functions is recommended [24]. AIN occurs most commonly during the initial year of therapy and it is non-dose-dependent. But in some patients with inflammatory bowel disease, AIN may occur as a complication of the disease [5].

### 4.4 Proton pump inhibitors (PPIs)

Proton pump inhibitors are used to treat acid-related gastrointestinal disorders. According to recent studies, many side effects of proton pump inhibitors have been reported. One of the side effects of the drug is nephrotoxicity, especially acute interstitial nephritis. PPI is thought to be associated with increased chronic kidney disease and its progression [5].

Recently, more concerns have been raised for proton pump inhibitors about the risks of acute interstitial nephritis, chronic kidney disease, and end-stage renal disease, and similar adverse kidney effects, such as interstitial nephritis and acute renal failure, have been attributed to histamine-2 receptor antagonists [26]. But according to a newly published review, these potential adverse effects of PPIs must be proven by demonstrable evidence [27].

### 4.5 Interferon (IFN)

Interferons are cytokines that protect body against viral infections. Exogenous interferons are used to treat hepatitis B, hepatitis C and various malignancies (IFN-$\alpha$), multiple sclerosis (IFN-$\beta$), and chronic granulomatous disease and malignant osteoporosis (IFN-$\gamma$). They may cause nephrotic syndrome with histological finding of minimal change disease (MCD), focal segmental glomerulosclerosis (FSGS) [5, 28, 29], and renal vascular injury [28].

### 4.6 Bisphosphonates

Bisphosphonates are used to prevent bone absorption. The oral forms are used to treat osteoporosis and are thought to be nonnephrotoxic. But IV forms (pamidronate and zoledronic acid) can cause nephrotoxicity. Some reports reveal MCD and FSGS—not otherwise specified (FSGS-NOS) after pamidronate therapy and some reveal collapsing—FSGS (C-FSGS) after IV zoledronate therapy [5, 30]. According to some reports, zoledronic acid mainly leads to ATN [29]. The severity of nephrotoxicity depends on dosing, infusion time, and total number of infusion. Ibandronate is thought to be safe for kidneys [30].

### 4.7 Lithium

Lithium carbonate is generally used to treat bipolar disorder. It causes multiple renal side effects, most commonly nephrogenic diabetes insipidus. Acute lithium toxicity causes ATN. Chronic lithium toxicity occurs after more than 10 years of therapy and most commonly causes chronic tubulointerstitial nephritis with distal tubular cysts and sometimes secondary glomerulosclerosis. Lithium also causes nephrotic syndrome and histological findings of MCD or FSGS. Rarely it leads to end-stage renal disease secondary to lithium-associated chronic tubulointerstitial nephropathy. Lithium may also lead to renal tubular acidosis and hypercalcemia [5, 29, 31].

### 4.8 Antiangiogenesis drugs (AADs)

AADs are used for treatment of cancers and neovascular eye disorders such as diabetic retinopathy, macular degeneration, and retinal vein occlusion. They cause nephrotoxicity by endothelial cell injury and thrombotic microangiopathy (TMA) [5, 29]. Clinical manifestations of AAD-associated TMA are proteinuria and hypertension [29].

#### *4.8.1 Chemotherapeutic agents*

##### *4.8.1.1 Mitomycin-C*

Mitomycin-C is an alkylating agent used for treatment of malignancies. It can lead to TMA and AKI. AKI is dose-dependent, and the risk of TMA significantly increases with the cumulative doses of >60 mg [5, 29]. While TMA can occur during therapy, it usually occurs several week, average 75 days, after last dosage [29].

*4.8.1.2 Gemcitabine*

Gemcitabine is a pyrimidine antagonist that is used to treat a variety of malignancies. AKI is dose-dependent. Higher cumulative dose and prior exposure to other chemotherapeutic drugs increase the risk of TMA [5, 29]. AKI occurs almost in all patients treated with gemcitabine. TMA most commonly occurs weeks to months after initiation of therapy [29].

### 4.9 Oxymorphone-hydrochloride

Oral-extended release formulation of oxymorphone-hydrochloride is a long-acting opioid that is used to treat moderate to severe pain. Some data reveal AKI and TMA secondary to IV abuse of the drug [5, 32].

### 4.10 Levamisole

Levamisole has been used in treatment of pediatric nephrotic syndrome, colon cancer, inflammatory bowel disease, and rheumatoid arthritis. It was removed from the market due to agranulocytosis side effect. But it is still available in illegal form mixed with cocaine. Levamisole may cause antineutrophil cytoplasmic autoantibodies (ANCAs)-associated vasculitis (AAV) [5]. It may also rarely lead to hyponatremia, Wegener's granulomatosis, and renal failure [33].

Also antithyroid drugs such as propylthiouracil, carbimazole, and methimazole, and an antihypertensive drug hydralazine may lead to AAV [5].

### 4.11 Angiotensin-converting enzyme inhibitors (ACE-Is)

Captopril is an ACE inhibitor that is used for treatment of hypertension and proteinuria. Kaptopril may be the only ACE-I leading to nephrotic syndrome [5].

### 4.12 Anabolic androgenic steroids

Anabolic androgenic steroids like testosterone and illicitly used forms may lead to CKD [34].

### 4.13 TNF-α inhibitors

TNF-α inhibitors are biologic agents. Based on renal biopsy and clinical findings, glomerulonephritis associated with systemic vasculitis (GNSV), glomerulonephritis in lupus-like syndrome, and isolated autoimmune renal disorder are the subgroups of autoimmune renal diseases that may be caused by TNF-α inhibitors [5].

### 4.14 Gold salts

Gold compounds have been used for treatment of rheumatoid arthritis, psoriatic arthritis, and juvenile idiopathic arthritis. Because of side effects, low efficacy, and high cost, newer medications take place of gold salts. Parenteral use 0f gold leads to proteinuria, and gold-induced proteinuria is an indication of gold discontinuation. With oral gold therapy, proteinuria is rare. Renal pathology shows membranous glomerulonephritis. This may progress to nephrotic syndrome in patients continuing gold therapy [5, 35, 36].

### 4.15 Amphotericin-B

Amphotericin-B is an antifungal agent that is the choice in immunocompromised patients. It causes AKI via the tubular cell toxicity [1].

Amphotericin-B damages membrane integrity by causing pores and increases membrane permeability, and this leads to distal renal tubular acidosis [16]. Risk factors for nephrotoxicity are similar as any toxic nephropathy, but sodium deficiency is important especially in patients taking diuretic therapy [4]. Preventive procedures of amphotericin-B nephrotoxicity include saline hydration before and after drug administration, use of liposomal formulations, limiting the duration of therapy, and considering a continuous low-dose infusion over a 24 hours' period [1].

### 4.16 Calcineurin inhibitors

Cyclosporine and tacrolimus cause reversible AKI by inducing afferent and efferent arteriolar vasoconstrictions. Persistent injury can lead to interstitial fibrosis and glomerulosclerosis, and this leads to irreversible chronic nephrotoxicity. Tacrolimus may cause TMA [16, 37].

### 4.17 Cisplatin

Cisplatin may affect glomeruli and distal tubule, but it primarily affects proximal tubules. It leads to tubular necrosis or tubulointerstitial disease. It may increase serum creatinine and decrease GFR and lead to hypomagnesaemia, hyponatremia, hypocalcemia, and hypokalemia. When administered with hypertonic saline, cisplatin is better tolerated [1, 4, 16].

### 4.18 Cyclosporin-A

Cyclosporin-A leads to acute reversible and chronic irreversible nephrotoxicity. Acute reversible form is seen most commonly in renal transplant recipients and manifests as acute renal failure. Chronic form typically manifests after 1-year therapy. Clinical features are marked decline in glomerular filtration rate (GFR), hypertension, mild proteinuria, and rarely hematuria [4].

### 4.19 Ifosfamide

Ifosfamide is an analog of cyclophosphamide [16] and is used in the treatment of solid tumors in both children and adults [1] Cyclophosphamide is not nephrotoxic, but ifosfamide is toxic to the tubular cell. It prefers proximal tubular toxicity and leads to Fanconi's syndrome [1, 16]. It may also affect glomerulus and decreases GFR. These impairments may lead to clinical manifestations including hypophosphatemic rickets, proximal and distal renal tubular acidosis, diabetes insipidus, and hypokalemia [1].

### 4.20 Foscarnet

Foscarnet is used for treatment of resistant cytomegalovirus (CMV) infections. It causes acute interstitial nephritis and intratubular crystal formation. Foscarnet may chelate with calcium and cause hypocalcemia [16].

### 4.21 Methotrexate (MTX)

Methotrexate is an antiproliferative and immunomodulating agent that is widely used. Its high-dose regimen leads to AKI. It may cause cellular damage or crystal nephropathy. Hydration therapy and urine alkalinization can prevent the concentration of MTX to become too high in the tubules. Also toxic systemic concentrations caused by AKI can be prevented by leucovorin administered 24–48 hours after MTX [1].

### 4.22 mTOR inhibitors

mTOR inhibitors such as sirolimus or everolimus can worsen any significant underlying proteinuria in liver recipients with preexisting chronic renal disease [1].

### 4.23 Vancomycin

Vancomycin is an antimicrobial agent used in the treatment of Gram-positive infections. Vancomycin use is associated with nephrotoxicity. Nephrotoxicity range was as high as 50% in the past, but now it ranges about 1.0–42.6% by newer formulations. In addition to common nephrotoxicity risk factors, patients weight exceeding 101.4 kg, daily vancomycin dose over 4 g are also risk factors for vancomycin nephrotoxicity [38].

### 4.24 BRAF inhibitors

The selective BRAF inhibitors vemurafenib and dabrafenib are used to treat metastatic melanomas. There are no data reported dabrafenib use causing acute kidney injury, but there are a few case series with vemurafenib. The Food and Drug Administration Adverse Event Reporting System (FAERS) reports renal toxic effect of both agents. Vemurafenib appears more nephrotoxic than dabrafenib. Although not clear, they are thought to cause tubular interstitial injury with hypokalemia and hyponatremia [39].

### 4.25 Dekstran

Dekstrans are used for volume replacement therapy and may cause acute kidney injury. Therefore, fluid status and urine output should be monitored closely [39].

### 4.26 EDTA

It is a chelating agent used to get rid of iron from the body. It may produce toxic effect that may be fatal. Genitourinary effects of EDTA are nephrosis, nephrotoxicity, occult blood in urine, and proteinuria [40].

## 5. Contrast-induced nephropathy

Contrast-induced nephropathy is defined as an increase in serum Cr level of greater than 0.5 mg/dL or 25% over baseline during a period of 12–48 hours after contrast administration and the exclusion of other causes of AKI [2, 41].

Contrast agents generally lead to reversible AKI. Histopathologic evidence generally shows ATN. Compared with other types of ATN, contrast nephropathy is usually characterized by relatively rapid recovery of renal function. Most patients are nonoliguric. If occurs, oliguria occurs immediately after the procedure. Other manifestations of acute kidney injury, such as hyperkalemia, acidosis, and hyperphosphatemia, may be present. The urinary sediment may show classical findings of ATN. Proteinuria is absent or mild [41].

Underlying chronic renal disease, diabetes, and nephrotoxic medications predispose patients to renal injury from contrast. If IV contrast is necessary, patients can be pretreated with N-acetylcysteine (600 mg twice daily for two doses before study and after study) and alkalinized IV hydration (three ampules of 50 mEq sodium bicarbonate in 1000 mL $D_5W$ solution). In most cases, Cr usually starts to decline within 3–7 days. Dialysis is rarely required for contrast-induced AKI [37].

## 6. Crystal-induced nephropathy

Crystal nephropathies cause mechanical obstruction, local intrarenal inflammation, and tissue injury. There are three subgroups of crystal nephropathies: renal ischemic, tubular injury, and obstructive nephropathy [42].

Crystal-induced acute kidney injury commonly occurs following the administration of drugs or toxins that are poorly soluble or have metabolites that are poorly soluble in the urine [3, 43]. Especially in volume depletion status, glomerular ultrafiltrate can be enriched with minerals, proteins, or drug metabolites. Acute accumulation can induce a sudden onset of crystal formation leading to AKI, and long-term accumulation can lead to CKD [3, 42].

Patiens with drug- related crystal- induced AKI are usually asymptomatic. Kidney injury usually manifests with increased serum Cr, accompanying with hematuria, pyuria, and crystalluria. Crystal-induced AKI is generally reversible by discontinuation of the drug. It may rarely progress to CKD and dialysis may be required.

Risk factors for crystal-induced nephropathies are intravascular volume depletion, underlying kidney or liver disease, and metabolic disturbances that change urinary pH [3, 43].

### 6.1 Sulfonamide antibiotics

Sulfadiazine and sulfamethoxazole are relatively insoluble in acid urine. Alkalinization of urine to a pH > 7.15 increases sulfadiazine solubility.

### 6.2 Methotrexate

High-dose methotrexate can both precipitate in the tubules and cause direct tubular injury. Alkalinization of urine to a pH > 7 increases methotrexate solubility. Methotrexate-induced acute kidney injury is typically nonoliguric and often reversible.

### 6.3 Indinavir

It is a protease inhibitor used in the treatment of human immunodeficiency virus infection. Acidic urine pH (<6) increases indinavir solubility, but acidification of urine may be harmful; thus, it is not recommended.

### 6.4 Ciprofloxacin

It is a fluoroquinolone antibiotic and causes acute interstitial nephritis and crystal-induced nephropathy. Crystals precipitate in alkaline pH [43].

The other drugs that may lead to crystal-induced nephropathy are acyclovir; protease inhibitors such as indinavir, atazanavir; foskarnet; megadose vitamin C; orlistat; oral sodium phosphate; purgatives; triamterene; and high-dose amoxicillin [2, 3, 16, 43].

### 6.5 Acyclovir

It is used in the treatment of herpes infections and sepsis in neonates. It can most commonly lead to crystal-induced nephrotoxicity and also to nephrotoxicity by direct tubular injury [21].

## 7. Conclusion

Many drugs both prescribed or over-the counter have potential to cause kidney damage. Therefore, some basic items such as past medical history, age and weight of the patient, drug-related risk factors, and nephrotoxic drug combinations should be taken into consideration before starting the treatment. If a nephrotoxic drug use is mandatory, patients should be followed up closely and frequently with appropriate biomarkers. Basic renal functions should be evaluated before treatment. The early detection of drug-induced nephropathies and application of the appropriate treatment methods are critical, because many patients recover when the drug is discontinued.

## Author details

Azade Sari
Abdi Sutcu Vocational School of Health Services, Cukurova University, Adana, Turkey

*Address all correspondence to: azadesari@gmail.com

## References

[1] Faught LN, MJE G, Rieder M, Koren G. Drug-induced acute kidney injury in children. British Journal of Clinical Pharmacology. 2014;**80**:901-909. DOI: 10.1111/bcp.12554

[2] Sinert R, Peacock PR. Acute kidney injury. In: Tintinalli JE, Stapczynski JS, Ma AJ, Yealy DM, Mecklern GD, Cline DM, editors. Tintinalli's Emergency Medicine. 8th ed. New York: McGraw-Hill; 2016. pp. 575-581

[3] Perazella MA. Pharmacology behind common drug nephrotoxicities. Clinical Journal of the American Society of Nephrology. 2018;**13**:1897-1908. DOI: 10.2215/CJN.00150118

[4] Dhodi DK et al. Drug-induced nephrotoxicity. International Journal of Basic & Clinical Pharmacology. 2014;**3**(4):591-597. DOI: 10.5455/2319-2003.ijbcp20140826

[5] Paueksakon P, Fogo AB. Drug-induced nephropathies. Histopathology. 2017;**70**:94-108. DOI: 10.1111/his.13064

[6] Barreto EF, Rule AD, Voils SA, et al. Innovative use of novel biomarkers to improve the safety of renally eliminated and nephrotoxic medications. Pharmacotherapy. 2018;**38**(8):794-803. DOI: 10.1002/phar.2149

[7] Meer L, Moerland M, Cohen AF, Burggraaf J. Urinary kidney biomarkers for early detection of nephrotoxicity in clinical drug development. British Journal of Clinical Pharmacology. 2013;**77**(6):947-957. DOI: 10.1111/bcp.12282

[8] Wasung ME, Chawla LS, Madero M. Biomarkers of renal function, which and when? Clinica Chemica Acta. 2015;**438**:350-357. DOI: 10.1016/j.cca.2014.08.039

[9] Andreucci M, Faga T, Pisani A, et al. The ischemic/ nephrotoxic acute kidney injury and the use of renal biomarkers in clinical practice. European Journal of Internal Medicine. 2017;**39**:1-8. DOI: 10.1016/j.ejim.2016.12.001

[10] Nayeri H, Babaknejad N. Evaluation of novel biomarkers in nephrotoxicity. Biomarkers in Medicine. 2016;**10**(12):1209-1212. DOI: 10.2217/bmm-2016-0235

[11] Waring WS, Moonie A. Earlier recognition of nephrotoxicity using novel biomarkers of acute kidney injury. Clinical Toxicology (Philadelphia, PA). 2011;**49**(8):720-728. DOI: 10.3109/15563650.2011.615319

[12] Gobe GC, Coombes JS, Fassett RG, Endre ZH. Biomarkers of drug-induced acute kidney injury in the adult. Expert Opinion on Drug Metabolism & Toxicology. 2015;**11**(11):1683-1694. DOI: 10.1517/17425255.2015.1083011

[13] Huang JX, Blaskovich MA, Cooper MA. Cell-and biomarker-based assays for predicting nephrotoxicity. Expert Opinion on Drug Metabolism & Toxicology. 2014;**10**(12):1621-1635. DOI: 10.1517/17425255.2014.967681

[14] Hooper DC. Beta Lactam Antibiotics: Mechanism of Action and Resistance and Adverse Effects. 2017. Available from: https://www.uptodate.com/contents/beta-lactam-antibiotics-mechanism-of-action-and-resistance-and-adverse-effects [Accessed: October 27, 2018]

[15] Palevsky PM. Manifestations of and Risk Factors for Aminoglycoside Nephrotoxicity. 2017. Available from: https://www.uptodate.com/contents/manifestations-of-and-risk-factors-for-aminoglycoside-nephrotoxicity [Accessed: August 27, 2018]

[16] Hughes PJ. Pathophysiologic Mechanisms of Selected Types of

Nephrotoxicity. 2017. Available from: https://emedicine.medscape.com/article/1925868 [Accessed: September 13, 2018]

[17] Hooper DC. Polymyxins: An Overview. 2018. Available from: https://uptodate.com/contents/polymyxins [Accessed: October 22, 2018]

[18] Demirturk N, Demir S, Asci Z, Dogan N. Evaluation of renal functions in patients treated with colistin. Nobel Medicus. 2016;**12**(1):74-78

[19] Curhan GC. Clinical Manifestations and Diagnosis of Analgesic Nephropathy. 2018. Available from: https://uptodate.com/contents/clinical-manifestations-and-diagnosis-of-analgesic-nephropathy [Accessed: October 24, 2018]

[20] Curhan GC. Epidemiology and Pathogenesis of Analgesic-Related Chronic Kidney Disease. 2018. Available from: https://uptodate.com/contents/epidemiology-and-pathogenesis-of-analgesic-related-chronic-kidney-disease [Accessed: October 24, 2018]

[21] Hanna MH, Askenazi DJ, Selewski DT. Drug induced acute kidney injury in neonates. Current Opinion in Pediatrics. 2016;**28**(2):180-187. DOI: 10.1097/MOP.0000000000000311

[22] Traub SJ. Acetaminophen (Paracetamol) Poisoning in Adults: Pathophysiology, Presentation and Diagnosis. 2017. Available from: https://uptodate.com/contents/acetaminophen-paracetamol-poisoning-in-adults-pathophysiology-presentation-and-diagnosis [Accessed: October 24, 2018]

[23] Acetaminophen (Paracetamol) Drug Information, Lexicomp. 2018. Available from: www.uptodate.com/contents/acetaminophen-paracetamol-drug-information [Accessed: October 24, 2018]

[24] Heap GA, So K, Weedon M, et al. Clinical features and HLA association of 5-aminosalicylate (5-ASA)-induced nephrotoxicity in inflammatory bowel disease. Journal of Chron's & Colitis. 2016:149-158. DOI: 10.1093/ecco.jcc/jjv219

[25] Chen J. Mesalamine induced nephrotoxicity in the treatment of crohn disease: A case study. Gastroenterology Nursing. 2014;**37**(1):70-73. DOI: 10.1097/SGA:0000000000000026

[26] Qiu T, Zhou J, Zhang C. Acid-suppressive drugs and risk of kidney disease: A systematic review and meta-analysis. Journal of Gastroenterology and Hepatology. 2018;**33**:1566-1573. DOI: 10.1111/jgh.14157

[27] Schubert ML. Adverse effects of proton pump inhibitors: Factor fake news? Current Opinion in Gastroenterology. 2018;**34**(6):451-457. DOI: 10.1097/MOG.0000000000000471

[28] Abudayyeh A, Perazella MA. Onconephrology: Kidney diseases in cancer patients. In: Comprehensive Clinical Nephrology. 6th ed. New York: Elsevier; 2019. pp. 776-785. ISBN: 978-0-323-47909-7. E-ISBN: 978-0-323-54719-2

[29] Markowitz GS, Bomback AS, Perazella MA. Drug induced glomerular disease: Direct cellular injury. Clinical Journal of the American Society of Nephrology. 2015;**10**:1291-1299. DOI: 10.2215/CJN.00860115

[30] Luedders DW, Steinhoff J, Thill M, et al. Lack of difference in acute nephrotoxicity of intravenous biphosphonates zoledronic acid and ibandronate in women with breast cancer and bone metastases. Anticancer Research. 2015;**35**:1797-1802. DOI: 0250-7005/2015

[31] Sterns RH. Renal Toxicity of Lithium. 2018. Available from: https://

uptodate.com/contents/renal-toxicity-of-lithium [Accessed: October 24, 2018]

[32] Hunt R, Yalamanoglu A, Tumlin J, et al. A mechanistic investigation of thrombotic microangiopathy associated with IV abuse of Opana ER. Blood. 2017;**129**(17):896-905. DOI: 10.1182/blood-2016-08-736579

[33] Brunt TB, van den Berg J, Pennings E, Venhuis B. Adverse effects of levamisole in cocain users: A review and risk assessment. Archives of Toxicology. 2017;**91**(6):2303-2313. DOI: 10.1007/s00204-017-1947-4

[34] Pendergraft WF, Herlitz LC, Brown DT, et al. Nephrotoxic effects of common and emerging drugs of abuse. Clinical Journal of the American Society of Nephrology. 2014;**9**(11):1996-2005. DOI: 10.2215/CJN.00360114

[35] Maini RN. Use of Gold Compounds in Rheumatic Diseases. 2017. Available from: https://uptodate.com/contents/use-of-gold-compounds-in-rheumatic-diseases [Accessed: October 24, 2018]

[36] Maini *N. major* Side Effects of Gold Therapy. 2017. Available from: https://www.uptodate.com/contents/major-side-effects-of-gold-therapy [Accessed: October 24, 2018]

[37] Mckenna BJ, Klintmalm GB. Postoperative intensive care management in adults. In: Busuttil RW, Klintman BG, editors. Transplantation of the Liver. 3rd ed. Philadelphia: Elsevier; 2015. pp. 866-894. DOI: 10.1016/B978-1-4557-0268-8.00069-5

[38] Meaney CJ, Hynicka LM, Tsoukleris MG. Vancomycin-associated nephrotoxicity in adult medicine patients: Incidence, outcomes and risk factors. Pharmacotherapy. 2014;**34**(7):653-661. DOI: 10.1002/phar.1423

[39] Jhaveri KD, Sakhiya V, Fishbane S. Nephrotoxicity of the BRAF inhibitors vemurafenib and dabrafenib. JAMA Oncology. 2015;**1**(8):1133-1134. DOI: 10.1001/jamaoncol.2015.1713

[40] Edetate Calcium Disodium (Calcium EDTA): Drug Information, Lexicomp. 2018. Available from: https://uptodate.com/contents/edetate-calcium-disodium-calcium-edta-drug-information [Accessed: October 22, 2018]

[41] Palevsky PM. Pathogenesis, Clinical Features, and Diagnosis of Contrast-Induced Nephropathy. 2017. Available from: https:www.uptodate.com/contents/pathogenesis-clinical-features-and-diagnosis-of-contrast-induced-nephropathy [Accessed: August 27, 2018]

[42] Palevsky PM. Crystal-Induced Acute Kidney Injury. 2018. Available from: https://uptodate.com/contents/crystal-induced-acute-kidney-injury [Accessed: September 11, 2018]

[43] Workeneh BT. Acute Kidney Injury. 2018. Available from: https://emedicine.medscape.com/article/243492-overview [Accessed: August 28, 2018]